the good food good mood

COOKBOOK

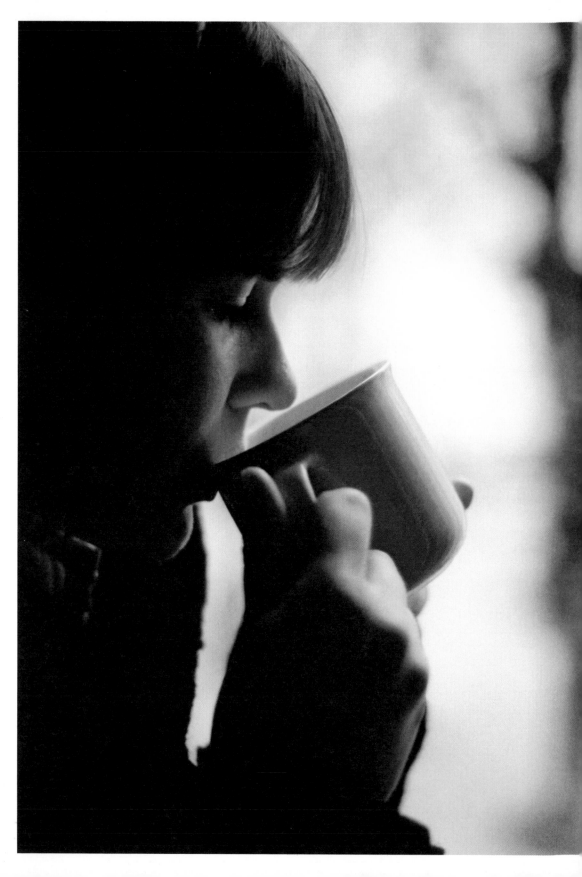

LINA BOU

the good food

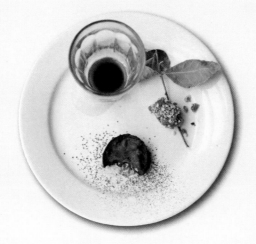

good mood
COOKBOOK

*Easy and healthy vegetarian recipes
for the modern lifestyle*

eddison
BOOKS LIMITED

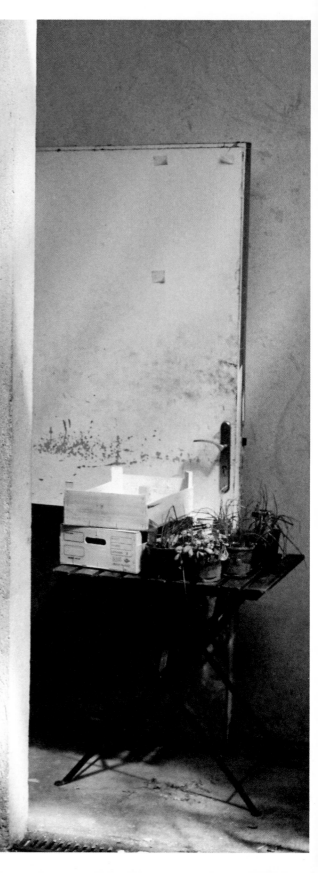

This edition published in Great Britain in 2018
by Eddison Books Limited
St Chad's House, 148 King's Cross Road,
London WC1X 9DH
www.eddisonbooks.com

British Library Cataloguing-in-Publication
data available on request.

ISBN 978-1-85906-410-8

10 9 8 7 6 5 4 3 2 1

Printed in China

Contents

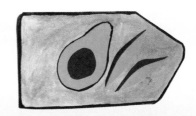

PREFACE

Hello! I am pleased to introduce you to my book, which I hope will not only inspire you to get some new ideas in the kitchen, eat more healthy food and learn more about herbs and holistic medicine, but also encourage you to experiment and invent new recipes to suit your own taste. Because that's what cooking is for me: no rules, no don'ts – and lots of fun.

My cookbook is for anyone who wants to be creative in the kitchen, enjoy life and have a healthy relationship with food. Good food is a huge part of life – but so is doing the things you love, like dancing, writing, practising yoga, exercising, playing music, travelling, spending time with friends and family … whatever it is for you. I want this book to be an inspiring tool, to broaden your mind and help you feel free and unrestricted, exploring new ideas to expand your culinary repertoire. I don't want you to forbid yourself from having certain foods, or feel guilty about eating something; what's important is to choose the foods that make you feel strong, healthy and happy. We all have our own, individual needs – and if you live your life with a positive mind and try to eat healthily, then that's something you can be proud of.

Because I want this book to be for everyone, most of the recipes are free from gluten, dairy and sugar, as, in my experience, these appear to be the most problematic ingredients when it comes to allergies and intolerances. Research shows that these foods can create inflammation in our bodies – and that we could avoid many diseases if we cut them from our modern diet. So, I want to inspire those who would like to explore this further in an easy way, because that's what cooking should be: easy, healthy and tasty. But don't worry – if you enjoy some sugar in your hot chocolate, or want to bake with butter, just do it! Some recipes also include suggestions for vegan alternatives, where possible, so there should be something for everyone here.

You will also see that each recipe features a health-category key, highlighting its benefits – so you can find out, at a glance, whether something is energizing, for example, or good for boosting your immunity, among other things (more about this on page 17).

My journey

As long as I remember, I've been interested in food and conscious of how it makes us feel. My passion for plants and herbs is largely down to my childhood years spent growing up in the idyllic countryside in Sweden, close to both forest and sea. To live in the natural world and see and smell the changes of seasons all year round, every day, fosters a greater sensitivity to nature, I believe. I have also been influenced by – and greatly admire – my Spanish aunt and uncle in Barcelona, who cook with such love and care for quality produce; they will spend hours making a wonderful paella with seafood from the harbour in town (or which my uncle has caught himself), and a broth that is so good it's like medicine for the soul. What inspires me is not just how simply they eat but how delicious the food is, always using local vegetables and meat, and how meals are always a precious time spent around the table (with some good wine!).

It wasn't until I went to see a nutritional therapist when I was sixteen years old, and started changing my diet and complementing it with natural medicine, that I saw and felt the huge difference. I was hooked. I was amazed to discover how clean foods, herbal medicine and your state of mind can change your life. I felt stronger and happier then ever before, and I wanted to know more about it and share this knowledge and natural tool with everyone! And this is where it all began …

I went on to study Herbal and Functional Medicine in Stockholm, and became a qualified nutritional therapist myself. Having worked in several health companies, with years of my own research and study under my belt, my website mytasteofhealth.com soon followed – and then came my dream of gathering together my knowledge in a book, along with answers to the questions I am most frequently asked … And here we are.

Let's have some fun!

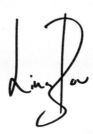

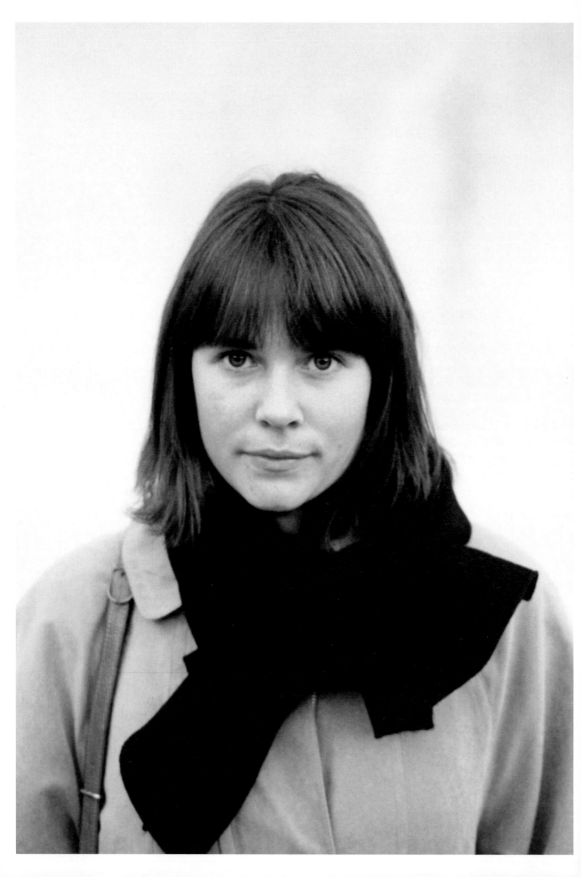

INTRODUCTION

A Brief 'Instruction Manual'

To give you a bit more information about what's going on inside your body, I've included a short instruction manual. This is a basic description of some of the very important functions performed by the body, which is an incredible, complex machine. It deserves more attention, but here I think a brief introduction is more than fair. So, there we go!

ENZYMES

Enzymes are our bodies' workers: like a house needs to be built using materials, with help from construction workers, the body needs to be built up with nutrition, helped by enzymes. More than 3,000 different enzymes have been identified, and each one has a different function. Enzymes drive the biological processes that are necessary for the body to build raw materials, circulate nutrients, eliminate unwanted chemicals, and the myriad other biochemical processes that go on without you even thinking about it.

What enzymes do:
Produce energy
Absorb oxygen
Fight infections and heal wounds
Reduce inflammation
Get nutrients into your cells
Carry away toxic waste
Break down fats in your blood, regulating cholesterol and triglyceride levels
Dissolve blood clots
Regulate hormones
Slow down the ageing process

Three different categories of enzyme:
Metabolic enzymes 'drive the body'. Needed for the building of new cells, they are everywhere, in our cells, organs and blood. All organs and tissues have their own enzymes. These enzymes are found inside the cells.
Digestive enzymes digest our food and break it down into smaller parts that can be absorbed, transported and utilized by every cell in our body. These enzymes are found outside the cells.
Food-based enzymes exist naturally in raw, uncooked food. When we heat our food to above 47°C (117°F), these enzymes are destroyed.

There are eight primary digestive enzymes, each designed to help break down different types of food:

Protease Digesting protein

Amylase Digesting carbohydrates

Lipase Digesting fats

Cellulase Breaking down fibre

Maltase Converting complex sugars from grains into glucose

Lactase Digesting milk sugar (lactose) in dairy products

Phytase Helps with overall digestion, especially in producing the B vitamins

Sucrase Digesting most sugars

THE DIGESTION PROCESS

Digestion begins in the mouth, where enzymes (primarily amylase) begin to exert their action. Here, amylase begins to break down carbohydrates. Once food has passed into the stomach via the oesophagus, protease gets to work on the proteins, breaking them down into amino acids. From there, the bolus of food passes into the small intestine, where 90 per cent of the digestion and absorption of food takes place. Here, lipase begins to break down fats and amylase finishes off the carbohydrates.

From here, the micronutrients are absorbed into your bloodstream, through millions of tiny villi (finger-like projections) in the wall of your gut. When this process goes wrong, diseases can occur; the root of many stomach problems is insufficient enzyme production.

The last 10 per cent of the digestion and absorption of food takes place in the gastrointestinal tract, stomach and large intestine. Water and electrolytes are absorbed in the colon, where the remaining waste material forms into faeces and is stored, before being expelled from the body via a bowel movement.

NERVOUS SYSTEM AND THE DIGESTION

Enteric nervous system (ENS)

One of the main divisions of the nervous system, the ENS consists of a mesh-like system of neurons that governs the function of the gastrointestinal system. It is usually referred to as separate from the ANS (see opposite), as it has its own independent reflex activity.

The ENS is often described as a 'second brain': it communicates with the central nervous system (CNS) through the parasympathetic and sympathetic nervous systems (for more on this, see page 169). It plays a role in the control of secretion of enzymes, and uses more than 30 neurotransmitters identical to the ones found in the CNS, such as dopamine and serotonin. More than 90 per cent of the body's serotonin is found in the gut, as well as about 50 per cent of the body's dopamine.

Autonomic nervous system (ANS)

The ANS is a division of the peripheral nervous system, which influences the function of internal organs. Our parasympathetic nervous system is responsible for the stimulation of the 'rest and digest' action that occurs when the body is at rest, especially after eating, including salivation, urination and digestion.

The sympathetic nervous system is another part of the ANS, and its action includes mobilizing our body's fight-or-flight response.

LIVER FUNCTION

The liver is the second-largest organ in the body, after your skin. Its job is to filter all the blood that comes from your digestive tract, thereby metabolizing nutrients, drugs, alcohol and other substances consumed while it detoxifies. It also manufactures proteins and produces bile, to help break down fats and clear bilirubin, a potentially harmful substance formed from the breakdown of dead red blood cells.

Liver and detox — why is it important?

A healthy liver will convert these harmful toxins into less harmful ones, or ensure they're eliminated from your body entirely. But some toxins get left behind, hiding in certain liver cells or creating free radicals (highly chemically reactive molecules) that can damage not just your liver but your overall health. It's therefore very important to support liver health in every way you can, by eating organic, sulphur-rich food, detoxifying your body regularly, exercising and consuming liver-supporting herbs (for more on detoxing, see pages 157–167).

NOTES ON INGREDIENTS

Superfoods

The following superfoods are so called because their nutritional compound is very high; some of them have been used for centuries and were considered to have medicinal properties.

Many of these ingredients have a long way to travel before they reach your home, so please consider this and use them sparingly. I do use these ingredients in my kitchen sometimes, and I love them for their benefits and unique flavours; however, I usually save them for special occasions, when I want to add that extra-special touch to a recipe.

Maca

- Maca is a plant from Peru. Its root is used in traditional medicine.
- Maca contains vitamin C, potassium, calcium and iron, among other essential vitamins and minerals. It's also high in protein.

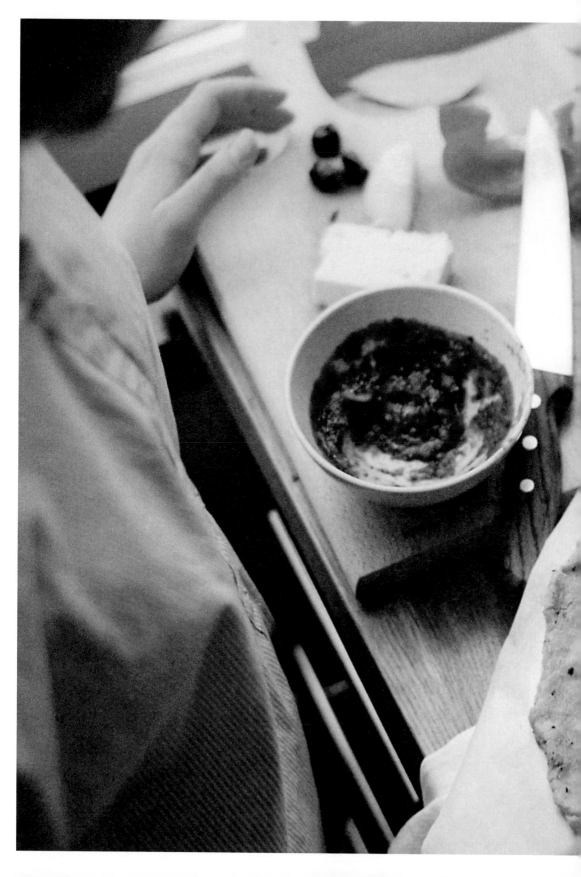

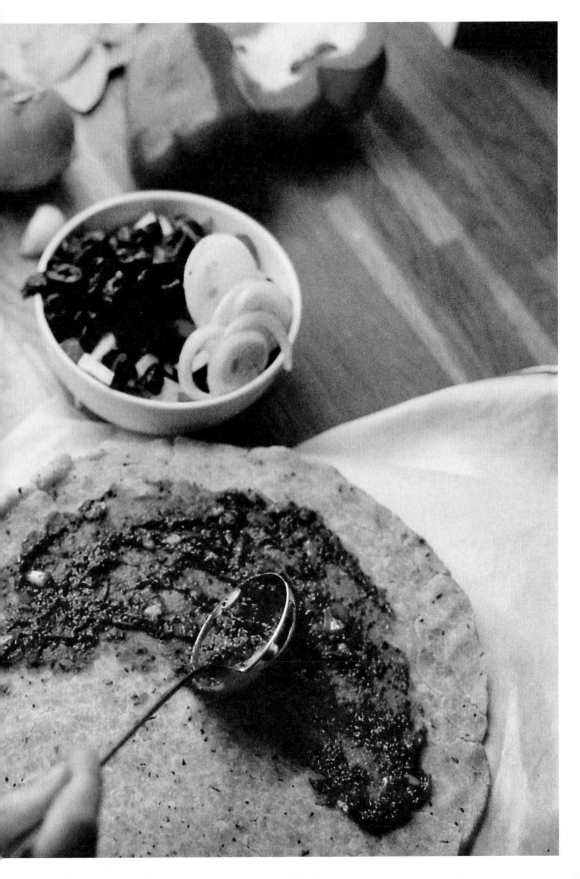

- Maca increases energy levels, boosts libido and sexual function and enhances fertility. It's also known for its ability to regulate the endocrine system, which affects hormonal balances.

Lucuma

- A sweet Peruvian fruit found in the Andes.
- Very rich in antioxidants, beta-carotene, iron, potassium, zinc, magnesium, calcium and phosphorus. It has a low glycemic index.
- Lucuma stabilizes blood sugar and gives long-lasting energy. Used for centuries in South America for its anti-inflammatory, anti-ageing and healing properties.

Spirulina

- A blue-green alga found in tropical salt water and some large freshwater lakes.
- High in protein, chlorophyll, iron, B vitamins and antioxidants.
- Spirulina is used for weight loss, improving digestion and bowel health. It helps to boost the production of white blood cells, which fight and prevent infection.
- Commonly used for its cleansing properties, detoxifying the body and cells of various heavy metals and toxins.

Chlorella

- A freshwater alga, originally grown in large, shallow and nutrient-rich freshwater ponds. Comes mostly from Japan and also China, Taiwan and India.
- Chlorella contains an enormous amount of chlorophyll (as the name suggests!) and is also rich in protein (about 58 per cent), B vitamins, vitamins C and E, amino acids and trace minerals.
- Contains nutrients required for many important biochemical functions, including hormonal balance. It has very good cleansing properties that remove heavy metals and other toxins from the body. It has been shown to boost the immune system, fight infection and balance blood pressure and cholesterol.

Chaga

- This wild mushroom is found on trees and grows in the birch forests of Russia, Korea, Eastern and Northern Europe and northern areas of the USA.
- Chaga is one of the richest sources of antioxidants in the natural world! It also contains vitamin K and calcium.
- It is considered a medicinal mushroom with anti-allergenic, antioxidant, skin-protective and adaptogenic qualities. It's commonly used as a medicine in China, Japan and South Korea.

Raw Cacao

- The cacao tree is native to the Amazon rainforest and also grows in tropical areas of North and South America, Africa and Asia. Each fruit contains about 25 cacao beans.
- It is a powerful antioxidant and contains phytochemicals such as flavanols, flavonoids, quercetin, caffeine and theobromine. It's also rich in many minerals, like magnesium, calcium and zinc.

- In Central America, the cacao bean is traditionally used to treat the pains of pregnancy, fevers and coughs. Theobromine is similar to caffeine but has less effect on the central nervous system. It is a stimulant that gives an energy boost, and it also relaxes the smooth muscle in the digestive tract.
- Cacao helps digestion and works as a mood-lifter, with its natural content of phenylethylamine and serotonin. It's also an aphrodisiac!

Chia

- Chia seeds can be used in baking as a natural thickener, as they swell and take on a special 'slimy' texture.
- According to internationally renowned natural health advocate Dr Mercola, black and white chia seeds contain similar amounts of omega-3s, protein and fibre, although the darker seeds may contain more antioxidants. To get the maximum benefit from chia, try to include both types in your diet.

SEASONAL EATING

A tomato salad in the winter is not at all the same as a tomato salad in the summer. You probably wouldn't enjoy eating a pineapple on a cold winter's day as much as you would on a hot day in summer. I do love things like coconut oil and avocado all year round, and I sometimes use superfoods from places like South America, but to support a sustainable environment and to get the highest nutritional value – not forgetting quality – it's best to choose food from your local farmers and producers.

As human beings living in a high-tech material world, where food produce is available all year round, we easily forget that we are part of nature. As the seasons, the climate and localized environment changes, the choice and availability of vegetables and plants are customized naturally. So, if we come from nature, doesn't it make sense that the vegetables and plants that are naturally best for us are those that grow close to us?

'Historically, nature, mountains, rivers, trees, the sun, the moon have always been honored in ancient cultures. It's only when we start moving away from our connection to nature and ourselves that we begin polluting and destroying the environment. We need to revive these attitudes that foster our connection with nature.' HUFFINGTON POST 16 July 2010

Eating locally grown and seasonal food is ultimately cheaper and better for small farmers, the community's economy and your pocket, and it also keeps us in step with the natural world. As individuals, we have an important role to play in this, supporting local farmers who manage their land sustainably.

Fruit and vegetables reach their nutritional peak around the time they are ready to harvest – and this is also when they taste best. For example, when tomatoes are at their reddest, they have their highest concentration of beta-carotene.

Winter might not be as sexy as summer, but have a look at all the winter goods you can enjoy (the list will vary slightly, depending on where you live):

Apples
Bay leaves
Beets
Broccoli
Broccoli rabe
Brussels sprouts
Burdock
Cabbage
Cardoons
Carrots
Cattail shoots
Cauliflower
Celeriac
Celery
Chestnuts
Chicory
Chickweed
Clementines
Collard greens
Cranberries
Cress
Endive
Escarole
Fennel
Frisée

Garlic
Garlic mustard
Grapefruit
Hazelnuts
Jerusalem artichokes
Kale
Kiwi
Kohlrabi
Lamb's lettuce
Leeks
Lemons
Lettuce
Limes
Mizuna
Mushrooms
Mustard greens
Nettles
Onions
Onion grass
Parsley root
Parsnips
Peanuts
Pears
Pecans
Persimmon

Pomegranates
Potatoes
Pumpkin seeds
Quince
Radicchio
Radishes
Rampion
Rocket
Rose hips
Rosemary
Sage
Salsify
Shallots
Sorrel
Spinach
Spring onions
Swede
Sweet potatoes
Swiss chard
Tangerines
Thyme
Turnips
Walnuts
Winter squash

And don't forget all the spices you can use all year round, without limits!

In the end, we are all nature.

HEALTH-CATEGORY KEY

Each recipe in the book – as well as being delicious and nutritious – also tells you *how* it's good for you, too. So, if you're after an energy boost, for instance, or something to help bolster your immune system, you can pick and choose your recipes accordingly. Look out for the category icons on the recipe pages (all recipes fall into at least one category, while some fall into two, three or even four – the 'superfood' equivalent of recipes!):

Digestion-friendly

Food that is easily digested, and which an upset stomach can handle, thanks either to digestive herbs, the cooking process or a combination of foods that are smooth and gentle on the digestive system.

Energizing

Recipes that leave you with a bit of extra energy thanks to the nutrients they contain or an energizing combination of ingredients. Great for a pick-me-up snack, or to enjoy before or after exercise.

Immunity-boosting

Dishes that boost your immune system due to containing a high amount of antioxidants and/or antibacterial properties.

Hormone-balancing

Food combinations that support a stable blood sugar and/or hormonal balance.

Fitness-building

This includes vegetarian recipes which have a source of vegetable protein, such as chia seeds, and foods that contain a good source of nutrients and protein to support the build-up of muscle tissue when exercising.

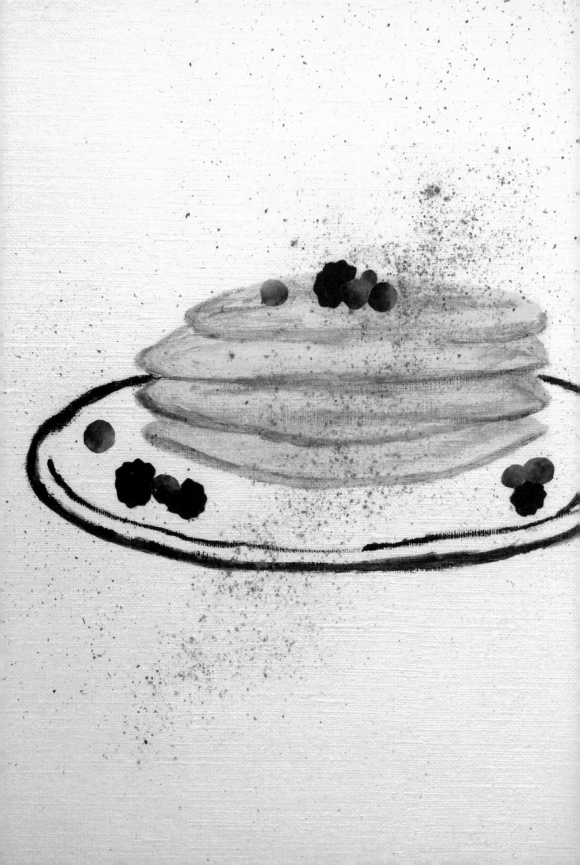

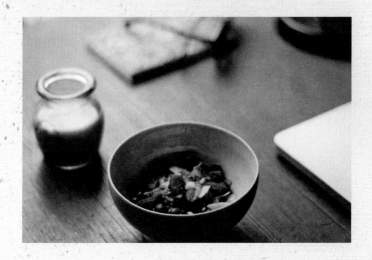

BRUNCH

The special thing about cooking is that you're creating something beautiful - nourishing your body and soul and giving yourself energy, to live.

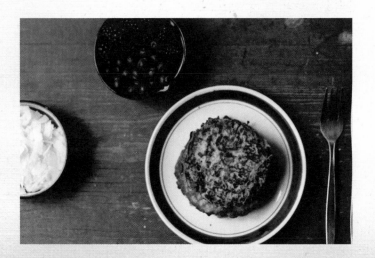

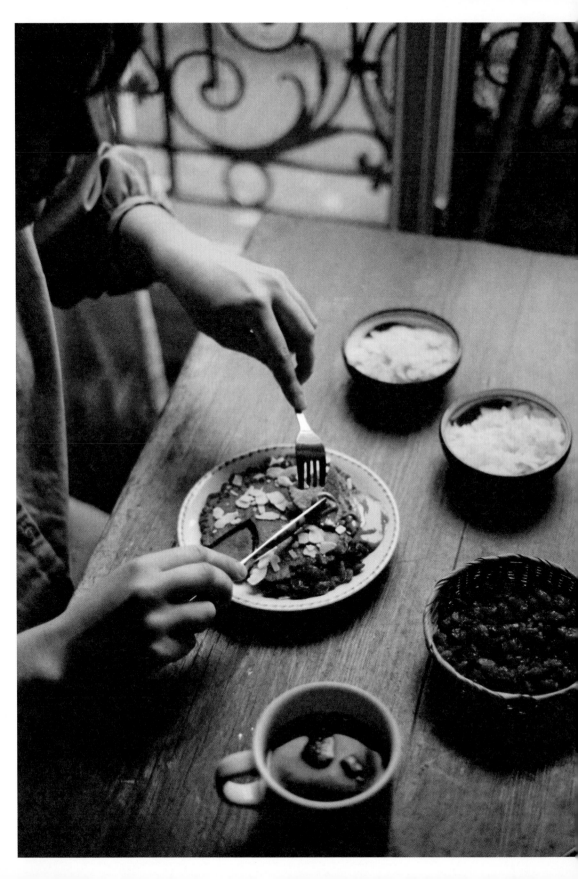

PANCAKES

BUCKWHEAT PANCAKES

120g (4¼oz) buckwheat flour
1 egg (vegan option: 1 tbsp flaxseeds and
3 tbsp almond milk)
150ml (5floz) oat, rice or almond milk
pinch of salt
extra virgin coconut oil (for cooking)

Makes 4 medium-sized pancakes

Mix together the flour and egg in a bowl, then add your choice of milk and the salt
and combine thoroughly with a whisk or fork. If you wish, you could add some
herbs or spices. Think about what you're serving your pancakes with when you
choose your flavours. For something sweet, maybe cinnamon or cardamom, or if
you're having your pancakes with salad and cheese, herbs like oregano, parsley
and thyme work well.

Heat some coconut oil in a frying pan and, when melted, pour about 2 tablespoons
of the pancake mixture into the pan and fry gently. After a couple of minutes,
when the underside is set, flip the pancake and cook the other side.

BEST BANANA PANCAKES

1 banana
50g (1¾oz) almond flour
1 tsp baking powder
1 egg (vegan option: 1 tbsp flaxseeds and
3 tbsp almond milk)
1 tsp ground cinnamon
pinch of salt
extra virgin coconut oil (for cooking)

Makes 3–4 medium-sized pancakes

Put the banana in a bowl and mash with a fork until the texture is creamy.
Add the rest of the ingredients and mix with a whisk or fork.

Heat some coconut oil in a frying pan, then add about 1½ tablespoons of the banana
mixture to the pan. Tilt the pan to spread the mixture over the base, then fry gently
on one side for a few minutes. When the underside is cooked, flip the pancake and
fry for a few more minutes to cook the other side.

Serve with coconut flakes, nut butter, cacao nibs, dried fruit or fresh fruit.
Be creative and enjoy!

Almonds are high in antioxidants that benefit the skin.

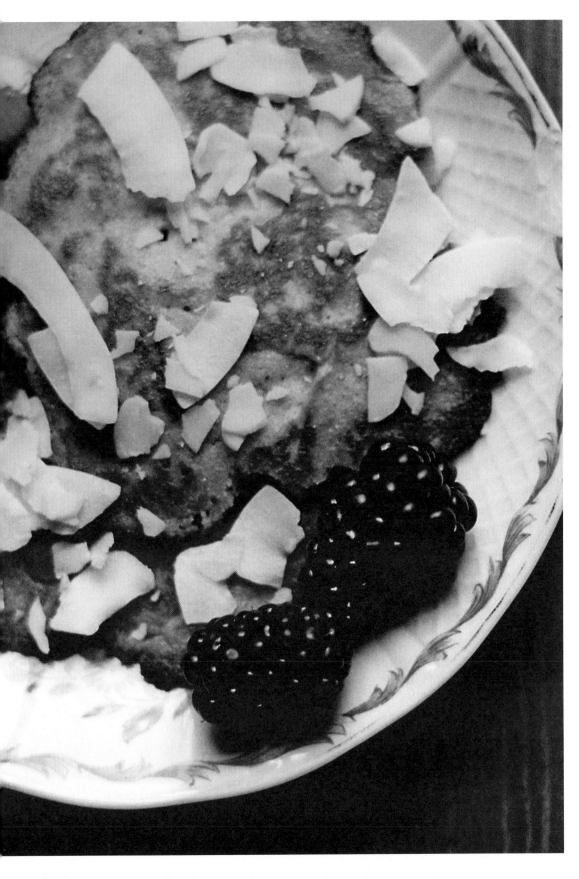

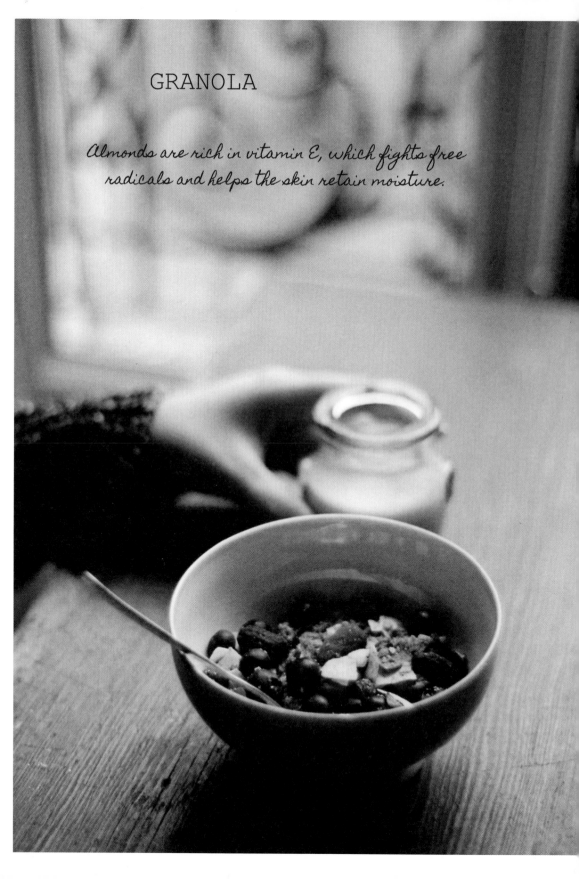

GRANOLA

Almonds are rich in vitamin E, which fights free radicals and helps the skin retain moisture.

EASY & QUICK GRANOLA

```
50g (1⅔oz) oat flakes
1 tbsp almonds
½ tbsp sunflower seeds
handful of coconut flakes
½ tsp ground cinnamon
1 tbsp honey (or agave syrup)
```

Serves 1

Put all the dry ingredients in a saucepan and heat for 5 minutes, stirring every now and then, until the mixture takes on a nice golden colour. Add the honey, then stir. The granola will now get crunchier, and in just a minute you'll have your own freshly made granola.

Serve with homemade milk (see below), or other milk of your choice, and some fresh berries or other fruit that's in season, for a very cheap, easy and fast breakfast. What a good start to the day!

ALMOND MILK

```
100g (3½oz) almonds
330ml (11floz) filtered water
```

Makes about half a litre of milk

Soak the almonds in the filtered water overnight. Strain and rinse the soaked almonds, then whizz in a blender.

Place a nut milk bag (see page 173) in a bowl, and empty the contents of the blender into the bag. Strain the yummy milk into the bowl. The almond meal will be left in the bag – you can use this in your scone or cracker recipes.

You don't have to use almonds; you can use other seeds or nuts with the same recipe – try sesame seeds, sunflower seeds, hemp seeds … Just add more water for a lighter milk, or less for a more creamy texture.

And why not also try vanilla almond milk? Just add 2 soaked pitted dates and 1 teaspoon of vanilla extract to the mixture.

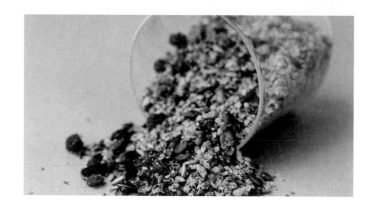

HOMEMADE GRANOLA

140g (5oz) buckwheat flakes
60g (2oz) almonds
70g (2¼ oz) sunflower seeds
30g (1oz) dried coconut flakes
35g (1¼oz) pumpkin seeds
½–1 tsp ground cinnamon
40g (1½oz) extra virgin coconut oil
¼ tsp ground vanilla
30g (1oz) honey (or agave syrup)
60g (2oz) dried mulberries, raisins,
figs or other dried fruit

Cinnamon is a super spice that improves digestion, balances blood-sugar levels and boosts metabolism!

Makes enough to fill one big jar

Preheat the oven to 180°C/350°F/Gas 4 and line a baking sheet with baking parchment.

Mix all the dry ingredients together in a large bowl.

Place a saucepan over a very low heat, add the coconut oil and honey and heat until melted. Add to the dry mixture and mix it all carefully with a spoon.

Spoon the mixture onto the prepared baking sheet and spread it out. Bake in the middle of the oven for 20–25 minutes, stirring it round a couple of times so it doesn't burn.

Place the baking sheet on a cooling rack to allow the granola to cool, before adding the dried fruit. Store in a glass jar.

Enjoy your fabulous breakfast!

CRUNCHY APPLE GRANOLA

210g (7½oz) buckwheat groats, soaked and sprouted (see below)
65g (2¼oz) almonds
75g (2½oz) sunflower seeds
50g (1¾oz) pumpkin seeds
¼ tsp ground vanilla
½ tsp ground cinnamon
2 apples, cut into small cubes
30g (1oz) honey (or agave syrup)
15g (½oz) extra virgin coconut oil
70g (2¼oz) coconut flakes
raisins (optional)

Makes enough to fill one big jar

Soak the buckwheat groats in water for 1 hour. Rinse, then leave under a towel for at least 24 hours, to allow them to sprout. This procedure makes the buckwheat more edible, as it's very hard, otherwise.

Preheat the oven to 175°C/350°F/Gas 4. Line a baking sheet with baking parchment.

Mix the buckwheat, almonds, sunflower seeds, pumpkin seeds, vanilla and cinnamon in a bowl, then add the apple cubes.

Place the mixture on the prepared baking sheet and pour over the honey and coconut oil. Gently combine, so that the honey and oil are evenly distributed. If you like your granola more sweet and moist, you could add up to another 20g (⅔ oz) of honey.

Bake in the centre of the oven for 30 minutes. During the second half of the cooking time, stir the granola every few minutes, so it is evenly cooked with a crunchy texture.

Remove from the oven and leave the baking sheet on a rack to cool, then add the coconut flakes and raisins (if using).

Soaking and sprouting the buckwheat activates the enzymes - it also makes it tastier and crunchier!

QUINOA GRANOLA WITH FIGS & CARDAMOM

100g (3½oz) quinoa flakes
35g (1¼oz) buckwheat flakes
80g (2¾oz) sunflower seeds
80g (2¾oz) almonds (whole or flaked)
35g (1¼oz) sesame seeds
2 tbsp extra virgin coconut oil
1 tsp ground cardamom
pinch of salt
4 dried figs, cut into small pieces
35g (1¼oz) coconut flakes

Makes enough to fill one big jar

Preheat the oven to 175°C/350°F/Gas 4. Line a baking sheet with baking parchment.

In a large bowl, mix together all the ingredients except for the dried figs and coconut flakes.

Spread out the mixture on the prepared baking sheet and bake in the centre of the oven for 20–30 minutes, stirring every 10 minutes, until nicely golden.

Leave the baking sheet on a rack to cool, then stir the dried figs and coconut flakes into the granola.

Quinoa promotes healthy intestines and gut!

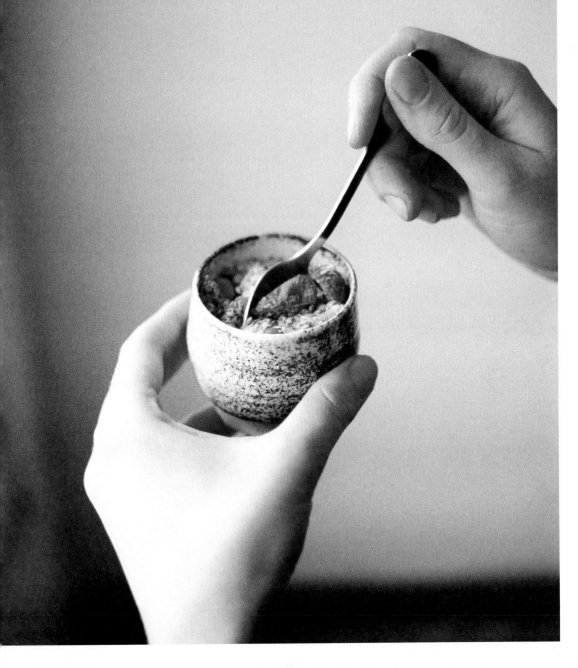

PORRIDGE

QUICK CRUNCHY MORNING PORRIDGE

60g (2oz) oat flakes
1 tbsp pumpkin seeds
½ tsp ground cinnamon
½ tsp ground cardamom
½ tsp ground nutmeg
1 cup of hot water
fruit and milk of your choice, to serve

Serves 1

Put the oats, seeds and spices in a saucepan and heat at a low temperature until the mixture turns golden.

Add a little of the hot water, stirring continuously. Add more water, a little at a time, until you get the texture you want. It should be crunchy.

Serve with any seasonal fruit and your choice of milk.

Breakfast is ready!

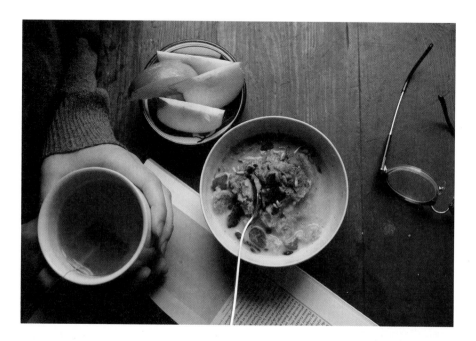

CHIA PORRIDGE WITH CACAO

Aztecs and Mayan warriors ate chia seeds – just a single tablespoon would keep them going for 24 hours. I like to use chia because it's very nutritious and produces a rich creamy texture. As an alternative, you can use flaxseeds or fibre husks, both of which have the same kind of effect.

1 tbsp chia seeds
90g (3¼oz) unsweetened almond milk
pinch of ground vanilla
1½ tbsp raw cacao powder
1 tbsp maca or mesquite powder (optional)

To serve:
Any seasonal fruit or berries
Mulberries
Cacao nibs

Serves 1

Put all the ingredients in a glass and stir with a spoon, then leave for 30 minutes.

Give the mixture another quick stir, then enjoy with some seasonal fruit or berries, mulberries and cacao nibs.

Chia seeds are high in protein and are perfect for breakfast, especially when you don't have much time but need that energy boost.

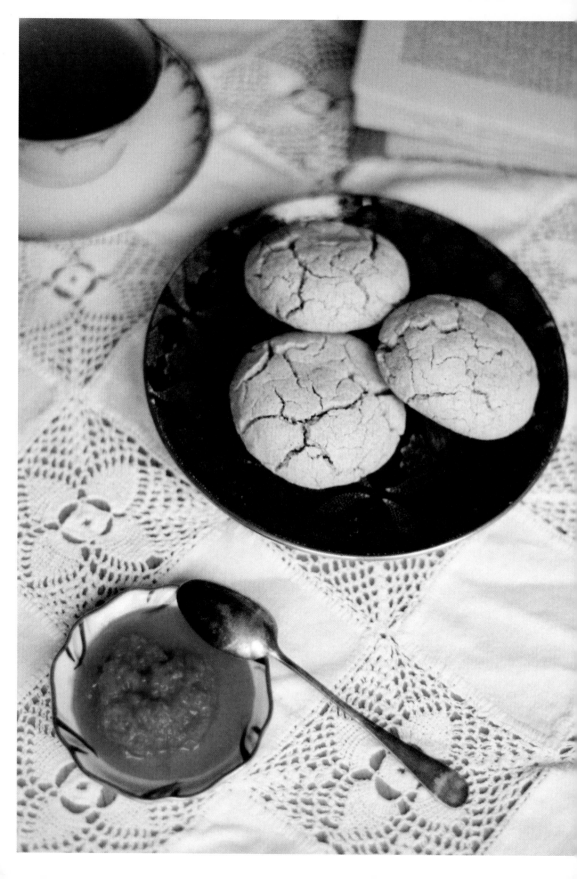

JAM

Do you always have a glut of berries at the end of the summer? Berry season is lovely, and sometimes, if you live in the countryside, you don't know what to do with all the berries and fruit that nature makes available. The best thing is to pick them and eat as much as you can fresh, and store the rest in the freezer. Another thing you could do is make your own berry purée or jam – and here's how.

RASPBERRY JAM

250g (9oz) raspberries
1 tbsp honey or maple syrup
1 tbsp lemon juice

Makes about 300g (11oz) of jam

Put all the ingredients in a saucepan over a low heat and bring to the boil, stirring continuously. Cover with a lid and simmer for about 10 minutes, until you have a purée consistency. Taste, adjusting the flavours if necessary, then leave the jam to cool. Store in a glass bowl in the fridge.

Serve on scones, with your granola or on top of your porridge.

Note that this is not a recipe to store over the winter; it's made to eat fresh, preferably within 5 days.

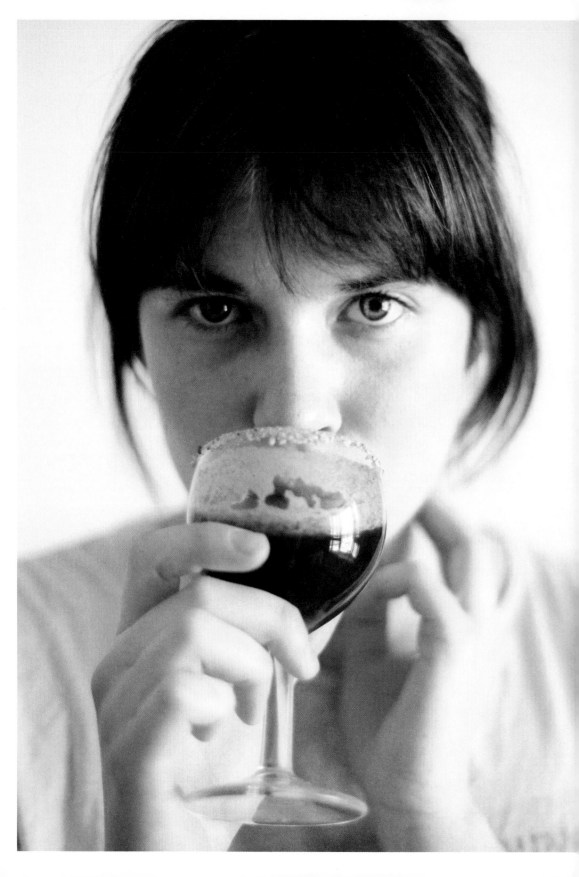

JUICES & SMOOTHIES

Smoothies and juices are a good option for when you're on the run, want a good start in the morning but don't have a big appetite, or to drink after exercise. You can reach a high level of nutrition in one smoothie or juice, thanks to being able to put many different vegetables and fruits in one glass.

Juice

Many people struggle to consume a healthy quantity of vegetables in one day; having them in a fresh juice is a good way to make sure your body obtains a large amount of vitamins and minerals.

It's important to remember that an excess amount of sugar can be harmful for the body, and this includes fructose, which naturally exists in fruit. I prefer to eat the whole fruit or make salads, but a green juice for a person who never eats salad can make a big difference to their nutritional status. Make sure that the majority of your juices are loaded mostly with vegetables like spinach or parsley, which contain lots of chlorophyll.

Smoothies

Smoothies are more filling than juices, contain more fibre and can even be treated as a dessert. When I make a smoothie, I think:

Base Which fruit/vegetable? (for example, spinach)

Taste Do I want a sweet or savoury flavour? (for example, lemon or soaked dates)

Filling Do I want the smoothie to be very filling or just provide a light energy kick? (for example, mixing it with almond milk, filtered water or coconut water)

Spice Do I add a superfood or my favourite spice? I like to use spirulina, cacao, cinnamon or just a good vanilla.

Voilà!

To get a higher level of protein in your smoothie, add a tablespoon of a nut or seed butter. My favourite is almond. You can also use different powders, such as maca and spirulina (see also 'superfoods', pages 11–15).

Superfood smoothies

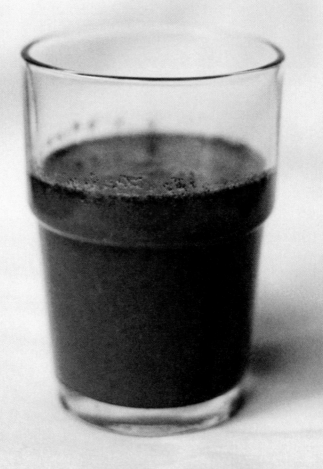

BERRY GREENS WITH BASIL

large handful of berries, frozen or fresh
(blueberries, raspberries or blackberries)
large handful of spinach
5 fresh basil leaves
1 tbsp almond butter
200ml (7floz) milk of your choice

Whizz all the ingredients together using a blender, and serve immediately.

Berries are a great source of powerful antioxidants. This is one of my favourite drinks, combining good protein, fibre, fat and chlorophyll – it's highly nutritious!

PROTEIN POWER SMOOTHIE

½ avocado
8 almonds (soaked overnight)
1 tsp chia seeds
1 tbsp raw cacao powder
1 tsp spirulina powder
filtered water (enough to achieve
your desired consistency)

Spirulina helps to boost the production of white blood cells, which fight and prevent infection.

Use a blender to whizz all the ingredients together, and enjoy – maybe with some granola on top!

CHOCO BANANA DREAM WITH MACA

1 ripe banana
1 tbsp maca powder
1 tbsp raw cacao powder
½ tsp ground cinnamon
½ tbsp almond butter
150ml (5floz) filtered water

Whizz all the ingredients in a blender, and serve. Add more water if you want a thinner texture.

A smooth drink that energizes and gives you vegetable protein – great for jetlag or before a workout.

Five juices

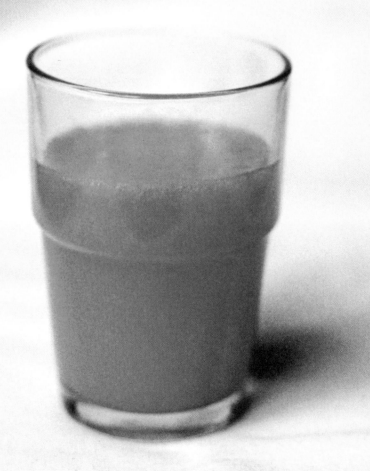

The following recipes are best made using a juicing machine or press. They each make enough for a big glass of juice.

FRESHEN-UP JUICE

This combination is diuretic and has a fresh and energizing taste. It supports the liver and is purifying.

```
2–4 celery stalks
handful of dandelion leaves
½ lemon
1cm (⅓in) piece fresh root ginger
1–2 pears
```

A juice that settles an upset stomach and helps the digestion.

TONIC JUICE

I'm not a fan of fruity juices, but grapefruit and blueberries are just the perfect combo of sweetness and bitterness and don't contain too much sugar. The three flavours in this recipe are great both for the taste buds and the digestion.

```
2 grapefruits
handful of blueberries
1cm (⅓in) piece fresh root ginger
```

Blueberries are beneficial for the eyes and rich in antioxidants.

THE GREEN JUICE

A green juice always feels fresh and purifying, and this one is very low in sugar.

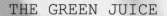

large handful of spinach leaves
1 tsp chlorella
1 lemon
1–2 apples

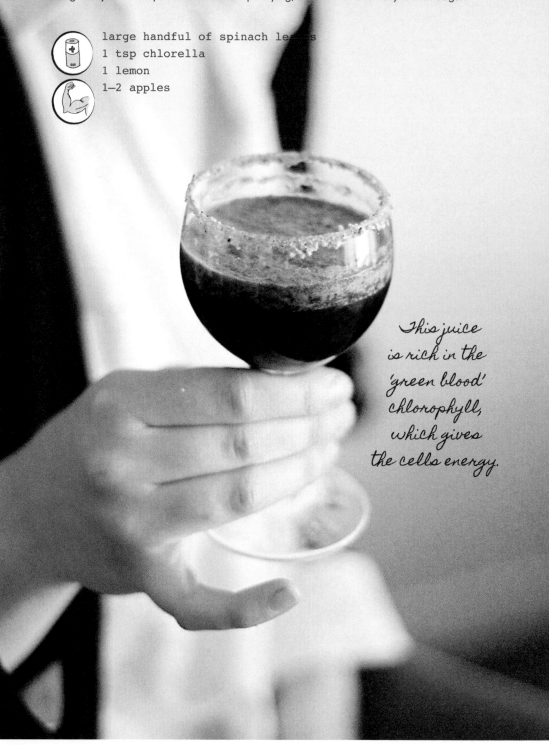

This juice is rich in the 'green blood' chlorophyll, which gives the cells energy.

CIRCULATION SPEEDER

I think cayenne and carrot go very well together in a juice, and, with the acidic touch of the lemon, are just balanced.

```
4–6 carrots
½ lemon
pinch of cayenne pepper
```

Cayenne is a strong anti-inflammatory spice, rich in vitamin C; it also gives you energy and helps blood circulation.

BLOOD PURIFIER

Pomegranate, one of my favourite fruits, contains a lot of vitamins, such as vitamin E, and it gives this juice a special taste and high nutritional status. The colour is beautiful; drink this after a night out, before or after sport or, maybe, as an aperitif before dinner with friends.

```
2–3 beetroots
½ lemon
seeds from ½ pomegranate
1cm (⅓in) piece fresh root ginger
```

Beets are rich in nitrates, which help to clean the blood.

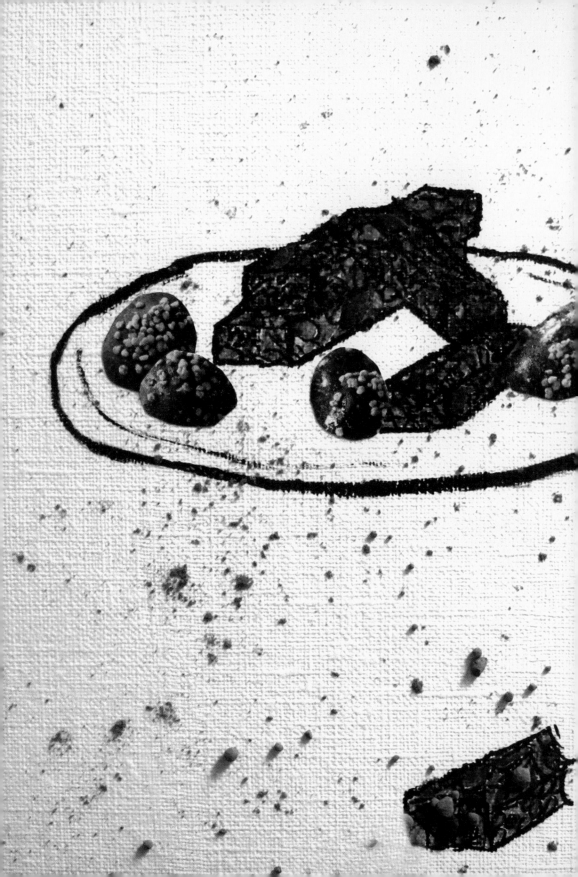

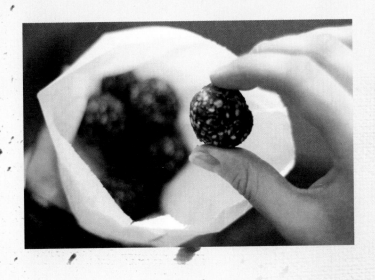

SNACKS

If you need energy on the run, rather than eating a big meal on the go, it's a better idea to have something like a juice, smoothie, a handful of nuts or one of these high-energy snacks, then eat something more substantial when you have time to sit down.

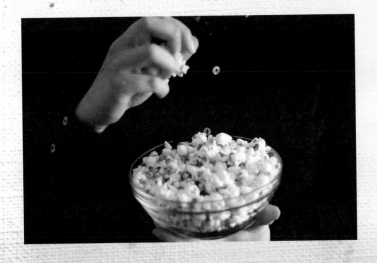

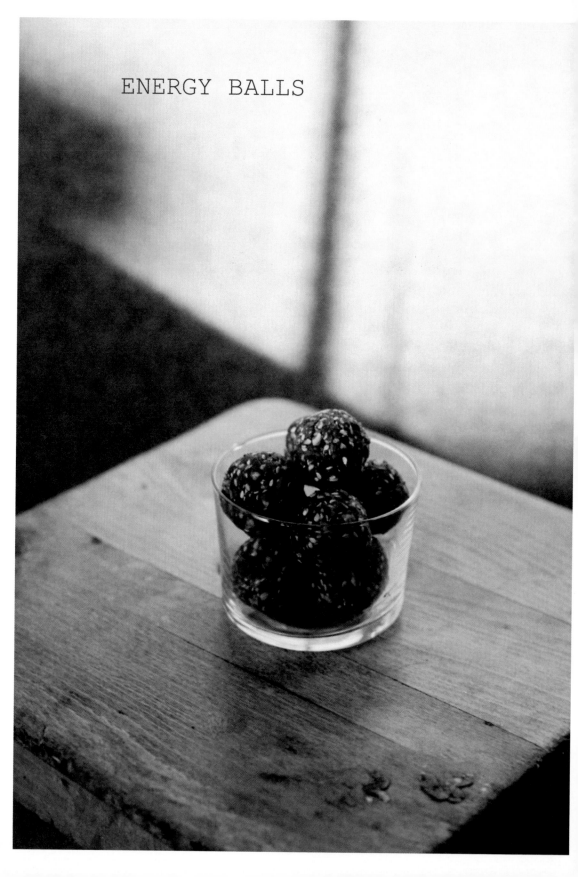

ENERGY BALLS

Mix and roll!

These energy balls are best kept in the fridge, where they will last for 4–5 days. If you're travelling around and keeping them at room temperature, they will be fine, but should be eaten within a couple of days.

CACAO & CHILLI CHOCOLATE BALLS

5 dates, soaked in water overnight or for at least 1 hour

65g (2¼oz) almonds

35g (1¼oz) sunflower seeds

30g (1oz) sesame seeds (or nuts such as cashews, hazelnuts, walnuts …)

3 tbsp raw cacao powder

pinch of cayenne pepper

pinch of salt

1 tsp water

Makes 15 balls

Remove the seeds from the soaked dates and discard. Put the dates in a blender, along with the rest of the ingredients, and whizz until well mixed.

Form the mixture into walnut-sized balls and store in the fridge until you're ready to snack!

In Central America, the cacao bean is a traditional remedy for the treatment of coughs and fevers.

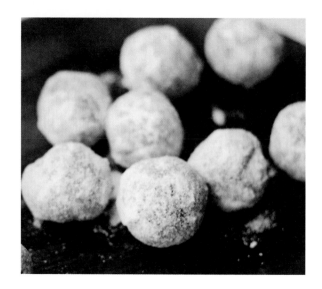

COCONUT BALLS

4 dried figs, soaked overnight or for at
least 1 hour
15g (½oz) coconut flour
35g (1¼oz) sunflower seeds
1 tbsp shredded coconut
2 tsp ground cardamom
pinch of salt
1 tsp extra virgin coconut oil, at room temperature
shredded coconut or coconut flour (for coating)

Makes 10 balls

Mix all the ingredients (except for the shredded coconut/coconut flour for coating)
in a food processor, along with about 1 teaspoon of water – just enough to allow
the blades to penetrate the mixture.

Using your hands, form the dough into walnut-sized balls and roll them in the
shredded coconut or coconut flour to coat. To get the balls nice and round, dust
your hands in coconut flour before rolling – this will make it easier and give you
a better shape.

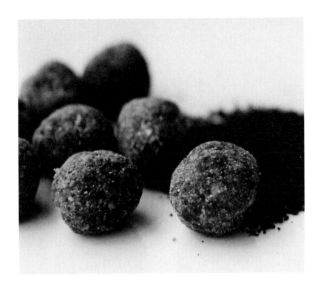

GREEN SUPERBALLS

65g (2¼oz) dried mulberries
juice of 1 lime, freshly squeezed
30g (1oz) pumpkin seeds
35g (1¼oz) sunflower seeds
20g (⅔oz) coconut flour
1 tsp spirulina powder
pinch of salt
1 tsp extra virgin coconut oil

Makes 12–14 balls

Put the dried mulberries and lime juice in a blender and whizz until well combined. Add the remaining ingredients and whizz again. When you have a good texture – not too finely ground, but without big pieces of seed – taste the mixture and adjust the flavours if necessary.

Using your hands, form the mixture into walnut-sized balls.

The blue-green alga spirulina is used to promote weight loss and also has cleansing properties.

CAROB TRUFFLES

125g (4½oz) almonds, soaked overnight or for at least 1 hour
2 large medjool dates, pitted
1 tsp carob powder
¼ tsp vanilla extract or ground vanilla
extra carob powder, for coating

Makes 13–15 truffles

Put the almonds and dates in a blender or food processor, together with a teaspoon of water, and whizz to combine. Add the carob powder and vanilla, then whizz again until the ingredients come together to form a ball.

Using your hands, form the dough into walnut-sized balls, then roll them in carob powder. Put the truffles in the fridge for 20 minutes before serving.

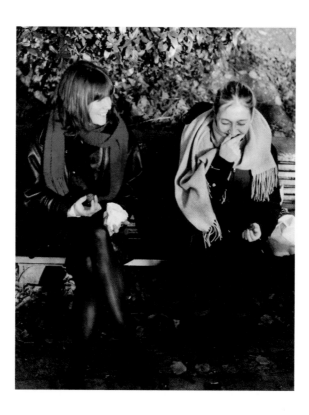

ENERGY BARS

THE ENERGY BITE

I used to make this recipe for a café in Paris and I want to share it with you here.
For me, this was the recipe I was missing whenever I went to a café for a good
snack and a coffee, but wanted something more filling and energizing than
a regular cake.

125g (4½oz) raisins
7 dates
190g (6½oz) almonds
75g (2½oz) pumpkin seeds
110g (scant 4oz) sunflower seeds
3 tbsp raw cacao powder
1 tbsp ground cinnamon
40ml (1⅓floz) warm water
sesame seeds or coconut flakes (to garnish)

*Contains lots of good
fibres, protein and
natural sweetener from
the dried fruits.
Yay!*

Makes about 15 bars

You will need a baking sheet measuring 30 x 20cm (12 x 8in). Line the tray with
baking parchment, leaving the edges overhanging (this makes it easier to lift out
the mixture later).

Soak the raisins and the dates for at least 1 hour.

Put the raisins, dates, almonds, pumpkin seeds, sunflower seeds, cacao and
cinnamon into a blender, then add some of the warm water (this will help the
blades to cut through the mixture) and mix until you have a pretty creamy,
but crunchy, texture.

Transfer the mixture into the prepared tray and use your hands to press it into the
corners. If you wish, you can place a small chopping board on top of the mixture
and press, to flatten. Sprinkle with the sesame seeds or coconut flakes, if using.

Chill it in the fridge for 1 hour.

Lift out the hardened mixture using the edges of the baking parchment, and cut
into bars using a sharp knife.

GRANOLA BARS

125g (4½oz) dates, soaked for 30 minutes
125g (4½oz) raisins
375g (13oz) almonds
1 tbsp almond butter
70g (2¼oz) pumpkin seeds
1 tsp ground cinnamon
extra virgin coconut oil (for greasing)

Makes about 15 bars

You will need a baking sheet measuring 30 x 20cm (12 x 8in).

Preheat the oven to 175°C/350°F/Gas 4. Grease the baking sheet with coconut oil and line with baking parchment, leaving the parchment hanging over the edges of the tray.

Deseed the soaked dates and put the dates in a food processor with a little water. Blend until you have a creamy mixture – this will bind the granola bars together.

Add the remaining ingredients, then pulse until you have a crunchy paste with some whole seeds still intact. You may want to add another drop or two of water, to help everything to mix together.

Transfer the mixture to the prepared tray and press it down well, so that it's flat with no gaps.

Put the tray in the middle of the oven and bake for about 30 minutes (all ovens vary, so keep an eye on the mixture, as it may not need quite this long). The granola bars should be a nice golden colour on the outside, but not burnt.

Place the tray on a rack to allow the granola to cool, then cut into 10 x 4cm (4 x 1½ in) rectangles.

Cinnamon is a strong antioxidant that boosts metabolism and gives you that extra energy. This is the perfect snack for when you're travelling!

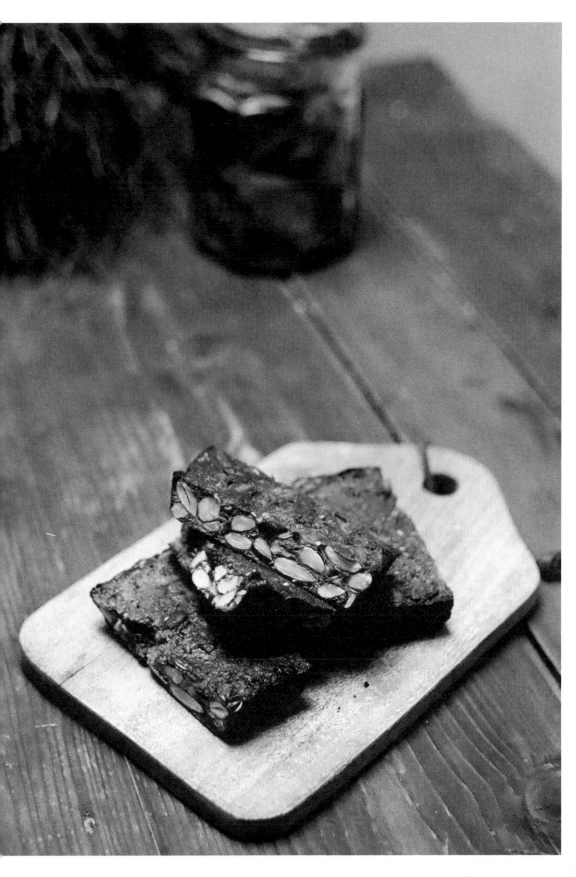

The cacao bean contains theobromine, a stimulant similar to caffeine but with less effect on the central nervous system.

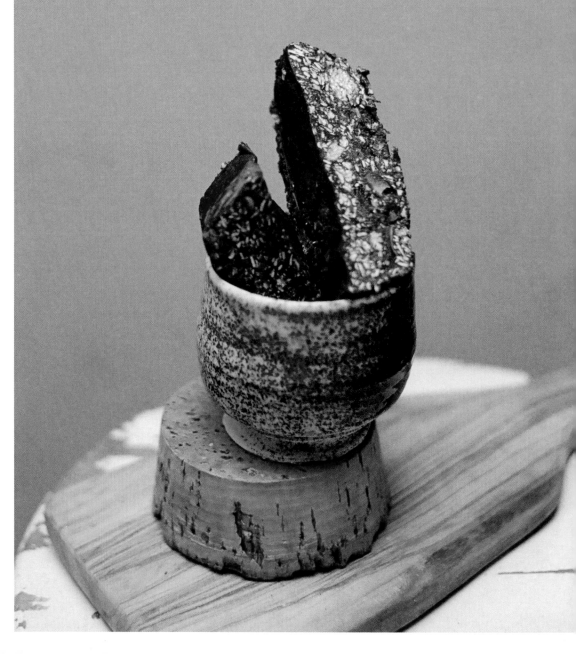

OAT BARS WITH CHOCOLATE

100g (3½oz) oat flakes
100g (3½oz) chocolate (made with 100% cacao)
100g (3½oz) dates (or any of your favourite dried
fruits, such as apricots, goji berries, cranberries …)
20g (⅔oz) sesame seeds

Makes 6–8 bars

You will need a 900g (2lb) loaf tin.

Preheat the oven to 175°C/350°F/Gas 4. Line the loaf tin with baking parchment, with the parchment hanging over the edges.

Spread out the oat flakes on a baking sheet and put them in the oven for 15 minutes, until they are nicely golden.

Melt the chocolate in a bowl set over boiling water (the bowl shouldn't touch the water).

Deseed the dates (or any other seeded dried fruit that you've opted to use), then chop them into small, thin pieces.

Using a mixer, combine the dried fruit with the oat flakes. Add the melted chocolate and mix well.

Transfer the mixture to the loaf tin, pressing it flat, and sprinkle the sesame seeds on top.

Put the tin in the fridge for at least 2 hours, until the mixture has hardened.

Lift the chocolate loaf from the tin, using the edges of the parchment, and cut into bars. They can be stored in the fridge for up to one week.

CRACKERS

FLAXSEED CRACKERS

50g (1¾oz) flaxseeds
100ml (3½floz) water
75g (2½oz) sunflower seeds
50g (1¾oz) pumpkin seeds
75g (2½oz) rice flour
1 tbsp extra virgin coconut oil
1 tsp sea salt
pinch of cayenne pepper (optional)
1 tsp cumin (optional)

Makes 9–10 crackers

Soak the flaxseeds in the water overnight, or for at least 2 hours.

Preheat the oven to 175°C/350°F/Gas 4.

Combine all the ingredients in a bowl. The texture should be creamy – not too wet, nor too dry.

Spread the mixture out on a baking sheet as thinly as possible, using a spatula – you may find it helpful to use your hands, too.

Using a knife, carefully score where you will cut the crackers (they should be about 10 x 15cm/4 x 6in), and bake in the middle of the oven for 30 minutes, until the crackers are thoroughly dried out, but not burnt.

Instead of cayenne pepper and cumin, you could experiment with other spices of your choice.

These crackers are a great accompaniment to many meals – and also handy when you're on the go. They are a good source of fibre and fill a hungry stomach in a comfortable and healthy way.

SPICY CHIA CRACKERS

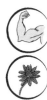

30g (1oz) chia seeds
250ml (9floz) water
50g (1¾oz) almond flour
100g (3½oz) quinoa flakes
30g (1oz) sesame seeds
20g (⅔oz) coconut flour
50g (1¾oz) cornflour
pinch of herbal salt
pinch of cayenne pepper

Makes 9–10 crackers

Soak the chia seeds in the water overnight, or for at least 1 hour.

Preheat the oven to 175°C/350°F/Gas 4 and grease a baking sheet.

Take your bowl of soaked chia seeds and add the remaining ingredients. When soaked, the seeds take on a creamy texture that will hold your crackers together. Mix everything together well.

With a spatula (along with your hands, if you find it helpful), carefully spread out the batter on the baking sheet as thinly as possible, and bake in the middle of the oven for 35–40 minutes. Halfway through cooking, turn the crackers over to allow them to cook evenly.

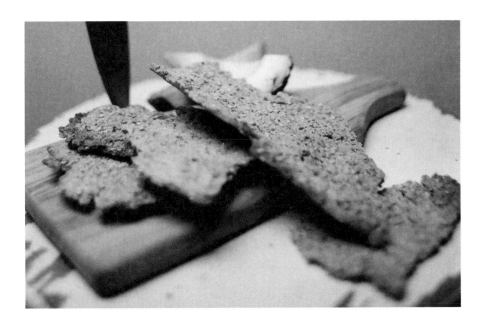

VEGGIE CRACKERS WITH VEGETABLE PULP

50g (1¾oz) flaxseeds
100ml (3½floz) water
70g (2¼oz) pulp from vegetables or fruits such
as carrot, apple, ginger, beetroot …)
80g (2¾oz) sunflower seeds
50g (1¾oz) buckwheat flour
1 tbsp extra virgin olive oil
1 tsp sea salt

Makes 9–10 crackers

Soak the flaxseeds in the water overnight, or for at least 1 hour.

Using a juicing machine, press your chosen fruit and vegetables and save the pulp –
the fibres that normally go in the compost.

Preheat the oven to 175°C/350°F/Gas 4. A convection oven will provide the best
results for this recipe.

Put the soaked flaxseeds in a bowl and add the pulp from the juicing process, then
the remaining ingredients. Mix together, then spread the mixture out on a baking
sheet, as thinly as possible.

Put the tray in the oven, on the middle shelf. After 15 minutes, when the mixture
has hardened a little, take the tray out and cut the crackers into squares. Return
the tray to the oven and continue to bake for another 20 minutes or so, until the
crackers are cooked, with a dry texture, but not burnt.

DRIED FRUIT & NUT MIXES

TRAIL MIX

```
50g (1¾oz) dried cranberries, non-sweetened
25g (⅞oz) cacao nibs
70g (2½oz) almonds
25g (⅞oz) sesame seeds
1 tsp chia seeds
```

Makes a small jar

Simply put all the ingredients in a jar and mix together. Keep it handy for those snacking needs!

Choose different nuts and seeds according to your taste.

This is a great source of protein and energy, for snack time and before or after sport.

TAMARI ROASTED ALMONDS

```
300g (11oz) almonds
2 tbsp tamari
spices of your choice, such as chilli powder
or ground cinnamon
```

Preheat the oven to 160°C/320°F/Gas 3.

Place the almonds on a baking sheet and pour over the tamari. Use your hands to mix the ingredients together and make sure the almonds are well coated.

Bake the almonds in the oven for about 15 minutes, until toasted.

POPCORN

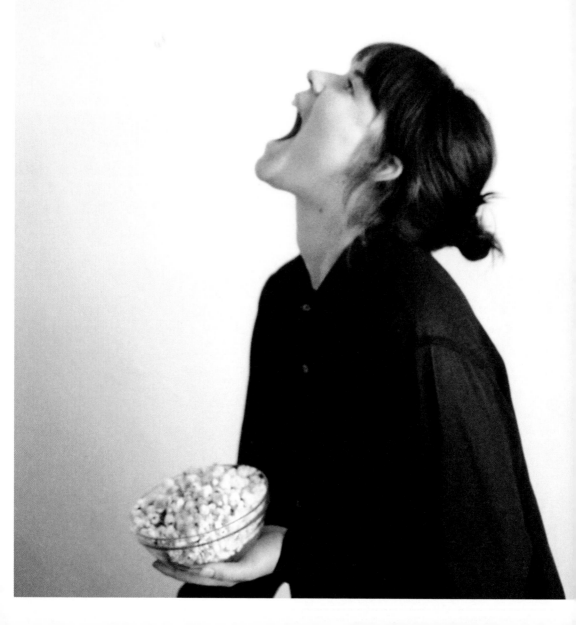

When I do my popcorn, I always use extra virgin coconut oil – first of all, I love the taste of coconut, but also because the oil can deal with high temperatures, up to 220°C/425°F, so it makes it a good oil for popping!

```
2 tbsp extra virgin coconut oil
250g (9oz) popping corn
flavour of your choice: classic salt or ground cinnamon,
lemon or cardamom — or why not chilli?
```

Heat the coconut oil in a saucepan over a high heat, then, when hot, add the popping corn and make sure you put the lid on. Once the corn starts to pop, give the saucepan a good shake every 30 seconds or so, to move the kernels around and prevent them from burning. It will take a while for the popping to start, but when it does it will get wild – don't be tempted to lift the lid!

When the popping starts to slow down, turn off the heat and continue to shake the pan every now and then until it's all quiet.

Pour the popcorn into a big bowl and add your chosen flavour.

Your popcorn is ready to eat!

MAINS & SIDES

Cooking for me is like when I paint or write. That is what I love, and I always work with colours as much as flavour combinations.

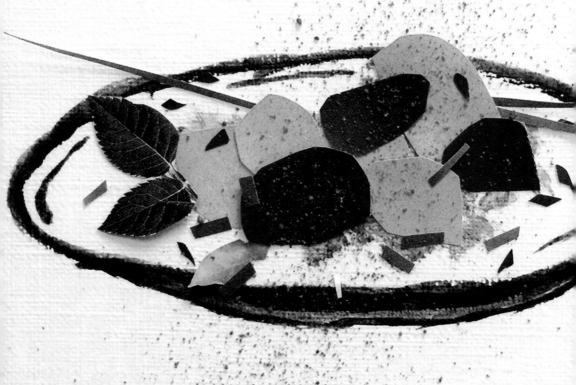

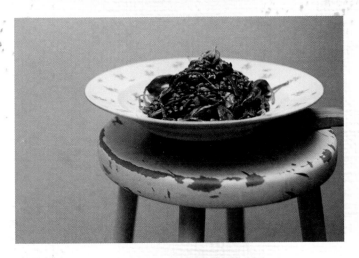

I like to use a variety of grains and seeds, as they all give you different vitamins and minerals, and mixing them gives you a more complete source of protein. Not only that, each vegetable colour has different nutrients – for example, dark green leafy vegetables such as kale, dandelion and spinach contain the carotenoid lutein, important for eye health. Just go to your local market and buy the fresh and seasonal vegetables that inspire you; each season and colourful vegetable has its charm.

Though I cook for a living, I am also pretty impatient and want dinner to be quick, and served in half an hour max most nights – especially when I've spent all day working in the kitchen. Still, I want to enjoy my meal, and I want to make it beautiful, but in a easy way – so I can assure you that the recipes are not too complicated.

I hope you enjoy them!

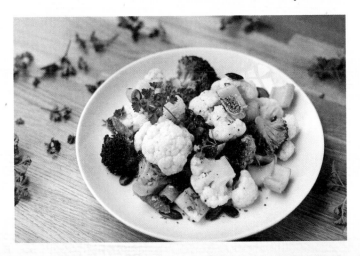

SIDES & SPREADS

Pesto

I love to make my own pesto; there are so many different flavour combinations to experiment with. I use whatever herbs I find at the market and mix them with what I have at home. I like to play with different seeds (raw or toasted) and oils like pumpkin seed oil and sesame oil. A pesto can pimp up a simple salad, be spread on crackers or combined with cooked lentils or beans.

Making a pesto doesn't take long. Once you've gathered the ingredients, just mix them together, then taste and adjust the flavours until you're happy with the balance. You can keep pestos for up to 5 days in the fridge.

Herbs like parsley, coriander and mint and other greens contain lots of chlorophyll, vitamins and minerals. The combination of the herbs with the healthy fatty acids and omegas in the oils and seeds gives pesto an even higher nutritional value, with more protein, fibres and fats – it will give you energy and a healthy glow.

Let's mix!

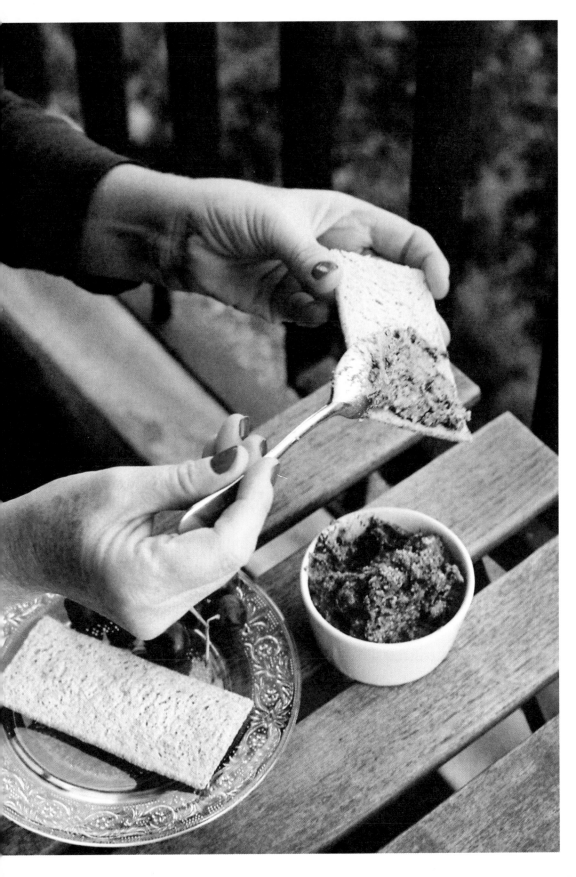

FRESH GREEN-LEAF PESTO

```
100g (3½oz) spinach
1 bunch fresh parsley
50g (1¾oz) sunflower seeds
45g (1½oz) extra virgin olive oil
juice of 1 lemon, freshly squeezed
salt and freshly ground black pepper
```

Makes enough for 1 medium-sized glass

Put all the ingredients in a food processor and whizz until everything is chopped thoroughly and well combined. You may need to add a little water if the blades get stuck.

This pesto works really well with the baked aubergine recipe on page 96.

Including leafy herbs in your diet is a great way to increase your daily antioxidant intake.

CORIANDER & PARSLEY PESTO

```
1 tbsp sunflower seeds
1 bunch fresh coriander
1 bunch fresh parsley
1 tbsp extra virgin olive oil
1 garlic clove, peeled
juice of ½ lemon, freshly squeezed
salt and freshly ground black pepper
```

Makes enough for 1 medium-sized glass

Heat a frying pan over a low temperature and add the sunflower seeds. Toast them, stirring occasionally, until golden. Leave to cool.

Put all the ingredients in a food processor and whizz until you have a creamy texture.

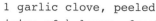

SPINACH & ALMOND PESTO

500g (1lb 2oz) spinach
100g (3½oz) almonds
2 tbsp extra virgin olive oil
juice of 1 lemon, freshly squeezed
salt and freshly ground black pepper

Makes enough for 1 medium-sized glass

Put all the ingredients in a food processor and blend to a nice texture.

Serve with crackers or a salad, as a dip or as you like it.

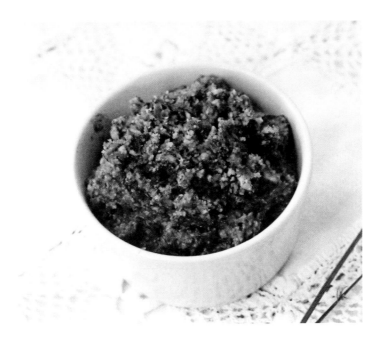

Spinach is a great source of essential minerals and vitamins, and studies have shown that it helps to maintain memory and mental clarity!

Pumpkin seeds are rich in essential minerals like magnesium and zinc, which are important for muscle strength, a healthy nervous system and intestinal health.

PUMPKIN SEED PESTO

100g (3½oz) pumpkin seeds
5 large basil leaves
2 tbsp freshly squeezed lemon juice
2 tbsp extra virgin olive oil
50ml (2floz) filtered water
½ tsp sea salt
½ tsp black pepper
1 garlic clove, peeled

Makes enough for 1 small glass

Preheat the oven to 175°C/350°F/Gas 4.

Spread out the pumpkin seeds on a baking sheet and toast in the oven for 10 minutes. Leave to cool.

Put all the ingredients in a food processor and blend until completely puréed.

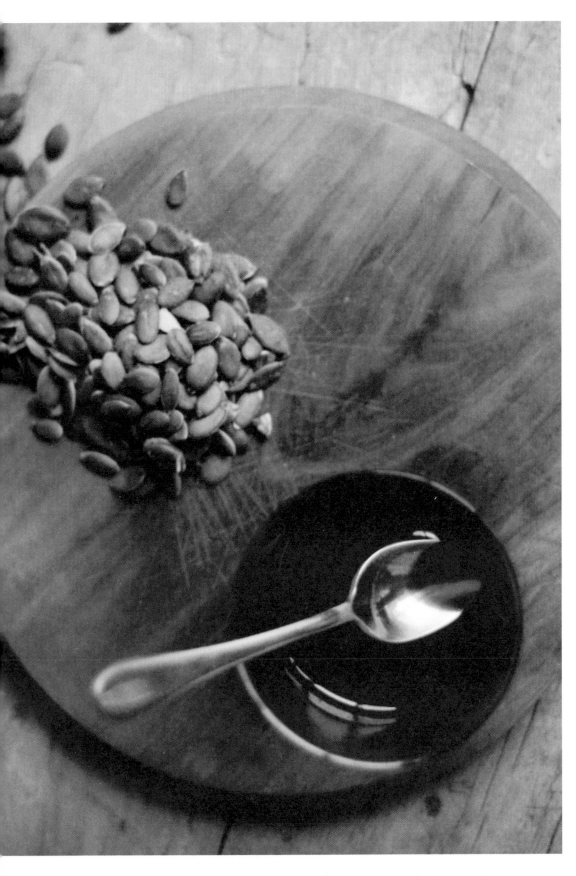

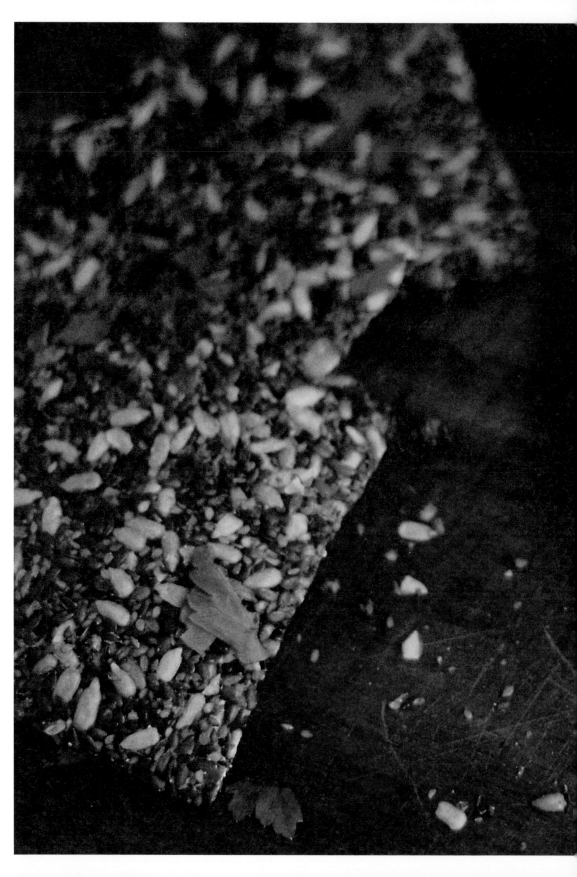

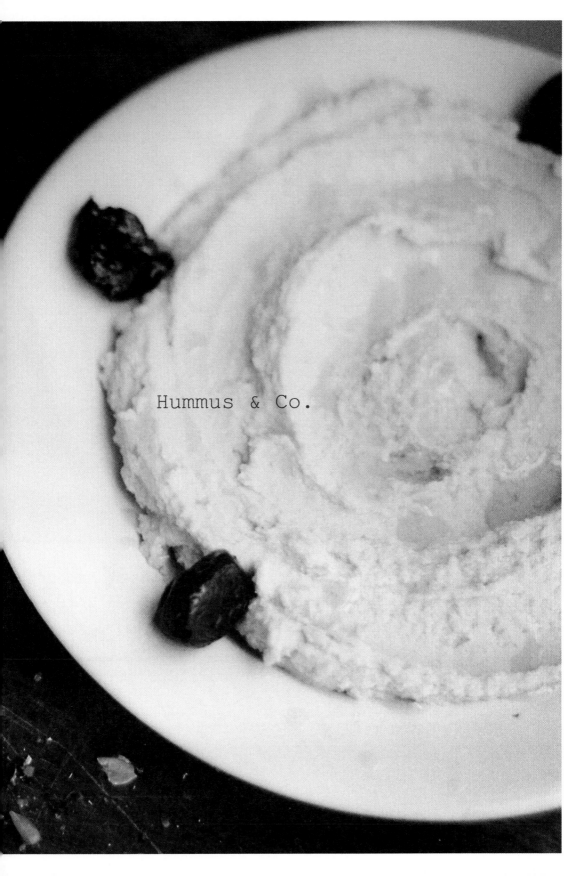
Hummus & Co.

HUMMUS

150g (5oz) dried chickpeas, cooked (see below)
1 tbsp tahini
2 tbsp freshly squeezed lemon juice
1 tsp sea salt
1 tsp freshly ground black pepper
2 tbsp extra virgin olive oil
1—2 tbsp water
handful of fresh coriander leaves
pinch of cayenne pepper (optional)

Serves 2 as part of a light meal, with a fresh salad and crackers, or serves
4–6 as a dip or spread

Rinse the chickpeas and put them in a blender, along with the remaining ingredients.
Add just enough water to enable the mixture to blend to a smooth texture.
Alternatively, you could use a hand mixer.

Serve with a drizzle of olive oil.

To cook your chickpeas:
You will get the best results if you use dried chickpeas and cook them yourself.
I always soak them overnight in water (using two times the volume of water to
the weight of the chickpeas, so if you have 150g/5oz of chickpeas, you'll need
300ml/½ pint of water), together with a teaspoon of baking powder. In the
morning, rinse the chickpeas and cook them in salted water over a low heat
for about 30 minutes, until softened.

*Chickpeas contain flavonoids and are a great source
of healthy fibres. Hummus is a tasty spread for
many occasions!*

SUPER GUACAMOLE

2 avocados
juice of ½ lemon, freshly squeezed
1 tsp spirulina powder
1 bunch fresh coriander, finely chopped
(plus an extra leaf, to garnish)
salt and freshly ground black pepper

Spirulina is rich in protein, chlorophyll and essential minerals. It boosts the nutritional value of your meal – but always use it raw, as heat destroys its vitamin and mineral compounds.

Serves 2

Put the flesh of the avocados, the lemon juice, spirulina powder (reserve a little to sprinkle on the top) and coriander in a bowl. Mash with a fork and season to taste.

Serve with a coriander leaf and sprinkle over the remaining spirulina.

FETA SPREAD WITH SUN-DRIED TOMATO & BASIL

5 sun-dried tomatoes, cut into small pieces
150g (5oz) feta cheese
3 tbsp freshly squeezed lemon juice
pinch of salt
freshly ground black pepper
5 fresh basil leaves, chopped
2 tbsp extra virgin olive oil

Makes enough for 1 small bowl

Put all the ingredients in a bowl and mash with a fork until you have the texture you want.

This makes a great accompaniment to salads, or a tasty spread to enjoy with crackers or bread.

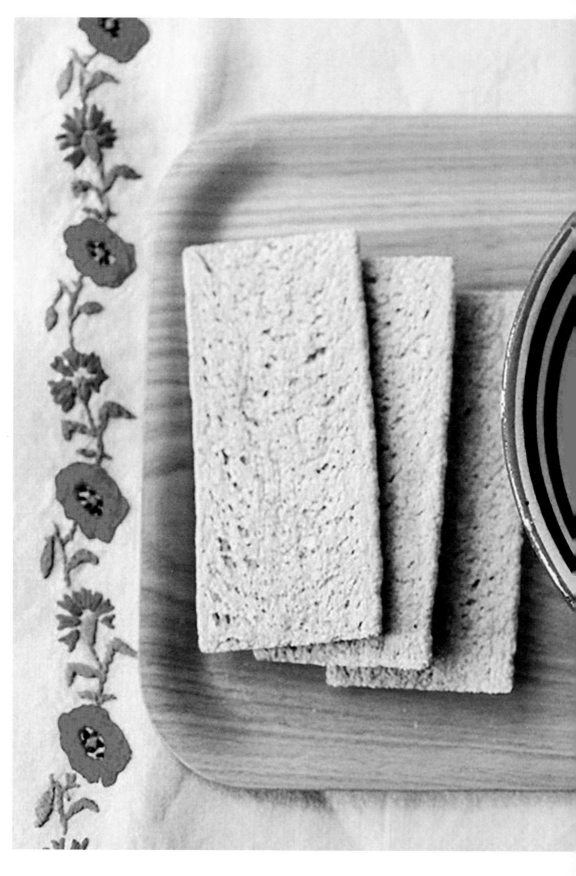

Spicy bean spread

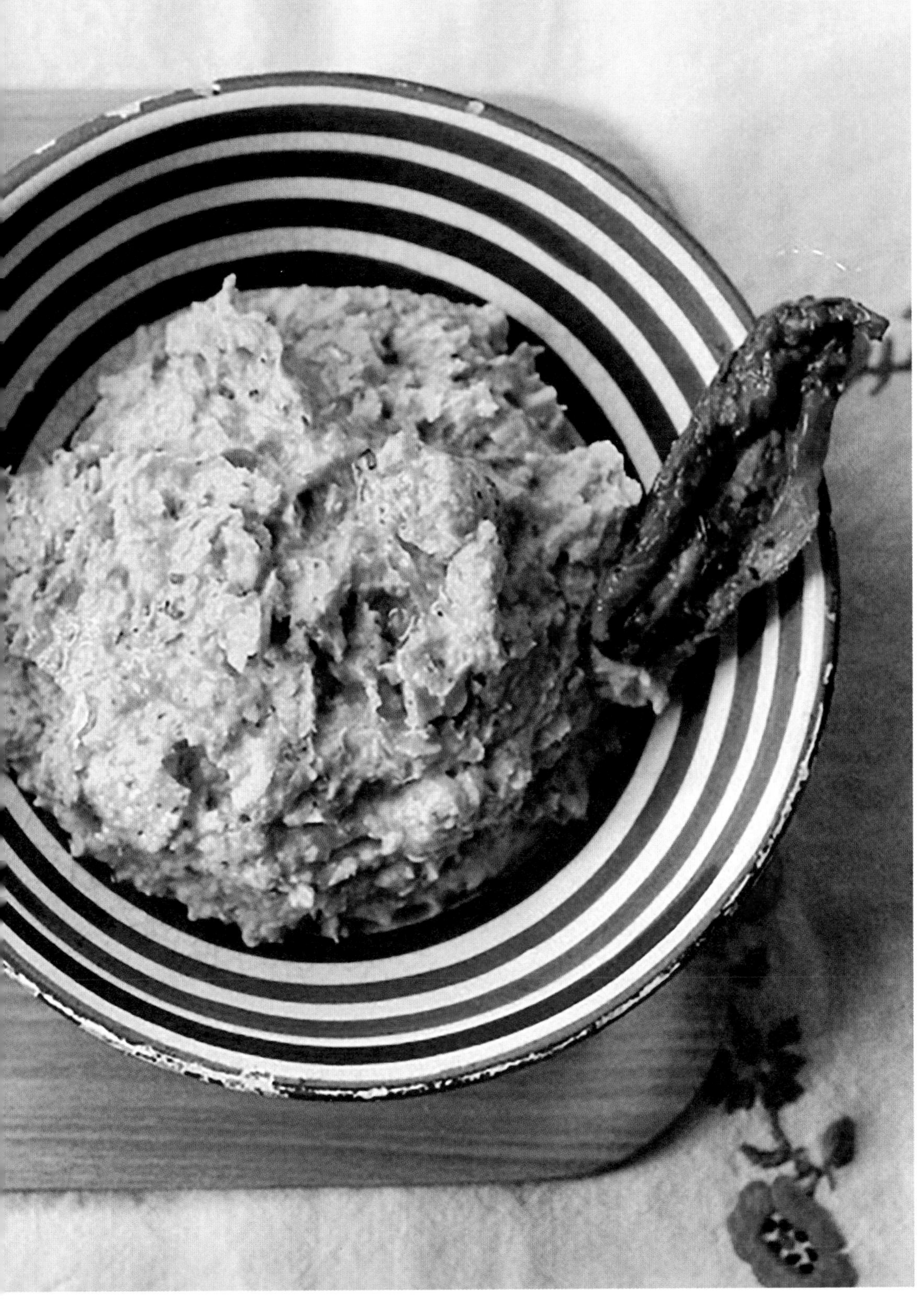

SPICY BEAN SPREAD

250g (9oz) white beans
6 sun-dried tomatoes
3 tbsp extra virgin olive oil
2 tsp chopped oregano leaves
pinch of chilli powder
2 tsp ground cumin
juice of ½ lemon
salt and freshly ground black pepper

Makes enough for 1 medium-sized bowl

Using a hand mixer or food processor, mix all the ingredients to a creamy spread.

This recipe goes really well with tacos. Serve with guacamole, some salsa and salad.

For a more Mexican touch, use black beans instead of white beans.

FRESH FETA SPREAD WITH GINGER & MINT

1 bunch rocket
2 tbsp freshly squeezed lemon juice
pinch of salt
150g (5oz) feta cheese
2 tbsp extra virgin olive oil
2 tbsp goat's milk yogurt (optional)
1cm (⅓in) piece fresh root ginger, finely grated
freshly ground black pepper
5 fresh mint leaves

Makes enough for 1 small bowl

Using your hands, mix the rocket with the lemon juice and salt, and let it marinate for a bit while you blend the feta cheese and oil in a mixer. If you want to make your spread extra creamy, add the yogurt.

Add the remaining ingredients and blend everything together until you have a nice creamy texture.

MY KIND OF GOMASHIO

3 tbsp sesame seeds (black and white are both good)
1 tbsp pumpkin seeds
2 sheets toasted nori seaweed
1 tsp sea salt

Makes enough to fill a small glass jar

Preheat the oven to 175°C/350°F/Gas 4.

Spread out the sesame and pumpkin seeds on a baking sheet and toast in the oven for 10 minutes. Leave to cool.

Break the nori into small pieces and grind using a Magic Bullet or KitchenAid (see page 173), until you have a very fine and powdery texture. (If you don't have access to either of these, use a pestle and mortar to grind the nori as finely as possible.) Add the toasted seeds and the salt, and mix on pulse mode until all the ingredients are combined and finely crushed.

SIMPLE SUPER VINAIGRETTE

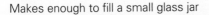

2 tbsp extra virgin olive oil
1 tbsp apple cider vinegar
1 tbsp lemon juice
pinch of herbal salt
pinch of black pepper
1cm (⅓in) piece fresh turmeric root, peeled
and finely grated (take care, as turmeric
stains very easily)

Serves 1

Mix all the ingredients together in a cup, using a whisk or a fork. Add straight to your salad and mix through, or place on your dinner table in a small glass jar and use as a side dressing.

MEALS

Hearty salads,
vegetables & grains

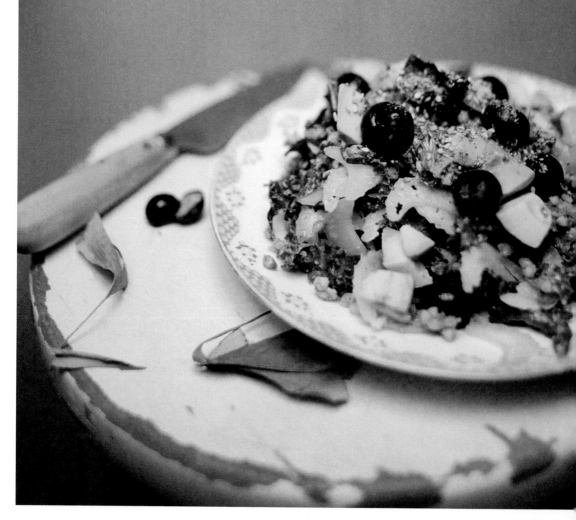

BUCKWHEAT TABBOULEH, GREEN KALE & BLUEBERRIES

1 tbsp extra virgin coconut oil
100g (3½oz) buckwheat groats
pinch of salt
300ml (½ pint) water
100g (3½oz) green kale, cut into small pieces
· 1 avocado
100g (3½oz) blueberries
4 sticks of celery, thinly sliced
25g (⅛oz) white sesame seeds

Sauce:
3 tbsp extra virgin olive oil
zest and juice of 1 lemon
1 tsp almond butter
salt and freshly ground black pepper

Serves 2–3

Heat the coconut oil in a saucepan, then add the buckwheat and salt and cook, stirring continuously, until the buckwheat turns golden. Add the water and bring to the boil, then simmer for 10–15 minutes, until the buckwheat is cooked to your liking – I like it a little al dente.

Meanwhile, in a large bowl prepare the sauce by simply combining the ingredients. Add the kale and, using your hands, toss it in the sauce so it's well coated.

Cut the flesh of the avocado into cubes and add to the bowl, together with the blueberries, celery and buckwheat. Sprinkle the sesame seeds on top. Ready!

Buckwheat has antioxidant and anti-inflammatory properties.

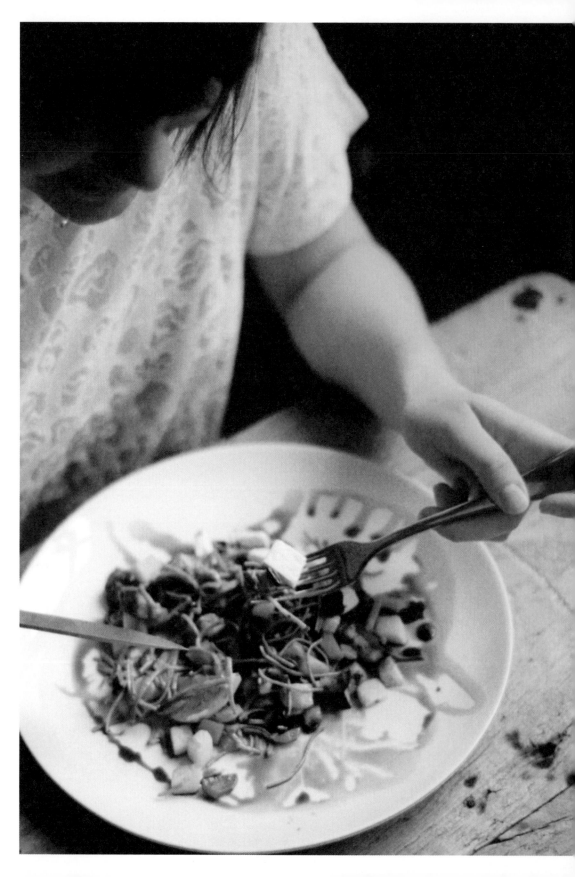

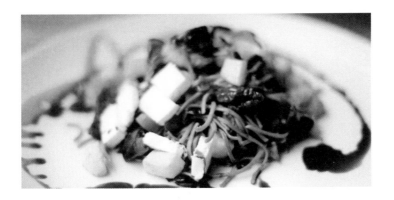

SOBA SALAD WITH ROASTED VEGETABLES & PUMPKIN SEEDS

1 packet soba (buckwheat) noodles
½ butternut squash, cut into small cubes
2 carrots, cut into small cubes
½ aubergine, cut into small cubes
35g (1¼oz) pumpkin seeds
coconut oil
salt and freshly ground black pepper
1cm (⅓in) piece fresh ginger, finely grated
1 bunch fresh coriander, rinsed
1–2 tbsp pumpkin seed oil

Serves 2

Preheat the oven to 175°C/350°F/Gas 4.

Cook the soba noodles according to the instructions on the packet, then rinse and set aside. Meanwhile, place the vegetables on a baking tray together with the pumpkin seeds and add some coconut oil, salt and pepper and the grated ginger. Mix thoroughly – ideally massaging the veggies with your hands – to make sure everything is well coated in the oil and seasoning. Bake in the oven for 30 minutes, or until the vegetables have turned a nice golden colour.

When the vegetables are done, add the cooked noodles to the tray and mix everything together, then put the tray back in the oven for 5–10 minutes to warm the noodles through. Take the leaves off the coriander stalks and add them to the salad, drizzle over the pumpkin seed oil and it's ready to serve. (For a tasty variation, try adding sun-dried tomatoes and a litte feta, too.)

The ginger adds a delicious spicy touch, as well as aiding digestion and giving your immune system a boost.

LENTIL SALAD WITH SEAWEED & TURMERIC

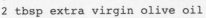

Turmeric is an antioxidant that fights inflammation – great for your immune system!

150g (5oz) green lentils

1–2cm piece fresh turmeric root, peeled and very finely grated (take care, as turmeric can stain very easily)

2 tbsp extra virgin olive oil

zest and juice of 1 lime (about 2 tbsp of juice)

salt and freshly ground black pepper

100g (3½oz) baby leaf spinach, chopped

1 avocado

30g (1oz) pumpkin seeds

20g (⅔oz) sea spaghetti

fresh parsley (to garnish)

Serves 2

Put 300ml (½ pint) of water in a saucepan and bring to the boil. Add the lentils and a pinch of salt. Cook gently for about 20 minutes, then rinse with cold water and set aside.

Put the grated turmeric in a bowl, together with the olive oil, lime zest and juice, salt and pepper and spinach. Cut the avocado flesh into cubes and add to the bowl, then add the lentils, pumpkin seeds and sea spaghetti.

Garnish with the parsley to serve.

OAT TABBOULEH WITH TAHINI SAUCE

1 tbsp extra virgin coconut oil
1 shallot, finely sliced
150g (5oz) oat groats
300ml (½ pint) water
handful of dried cranberries
50g (1¾oz) seasonal leafy greens
(e.g. spinach or rocket)
5 fresh sage leaves, roughly chopped
flat-leaf parsley (to garnish)

Sauce:
2 tbsp extra virgin olive oil
1 tbsp white tahini
2 tbsp freshly squeezed lemon juice
salt and freshly ground black pepper

Serves 2–3

Heat the coconut oil in a saucepan, then add the shallot and the oats, and cook
gently until they turn golden. Add enough water to cover the oats, then bring
to the boil and simmer gently, adding more water once the initial amount has
evaporated, 'risotto style'. Stir, then leave to simmer very gently for about
30 minutes, until al dente.

Meanwhile, prepare the sauce. Put all the ingredients in a bowl and mix with
a fork until well combined.

Add the tabbouleh to the sauce, then sprinkle over the dried cranberries,
greens, sage and parsley.

The botanical name for sage is 'Salvia', which comes from the Latin word 'salvere', meaning 'to heal' or 'to save'. Sage has antibacterial and anti-inflammatory properties and a great unique taste!

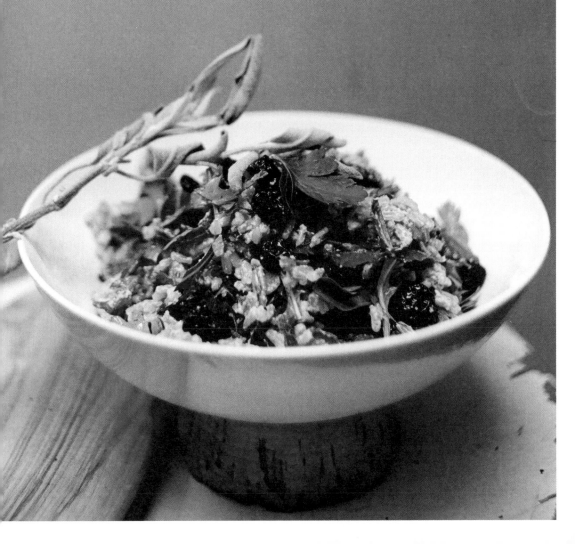

CHICKPEA SALAD WITH MUSTARD SAUCE

200g (7oz) green beans, topped and tailed
30g (1oz) sunflower seeds
1 bunch fresh parsley, chopped
1 bunch fresh coriander, chopped
1 tsp Dijon mustard
2 tbsp extra virgin olive oil
zest and juice of ½ lemon
250g (9oz) dried chickpeas, cooked (see page 70),
or 2 x 400g (14oz) can chickpeas
salt and freshly ground black pepper

Serves 4

Pour 1 litre (1¾ pints) of water into a saucepan and bring to the boil. Add the green beans and simmer for 7 minutes. When cooked, rinse with cold water, transfer to a bowl and set aside.

Heat a frying pan over a low heat and gently toast the sunflower seeds until they turn golden brown.

Take the bowl containing the green beans and add the mustard, olive oil and lemon zest and juice, then mix together with the chickpeas and some of the sunflower seeds, and season to taste.

Stir through the chopped parsley and coriander, and sprinkle over the remaining seeds to serve.

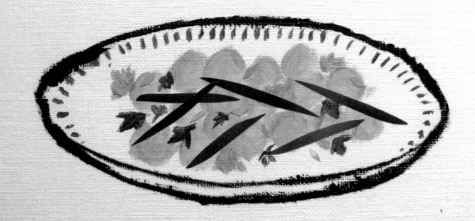

Fresh salads

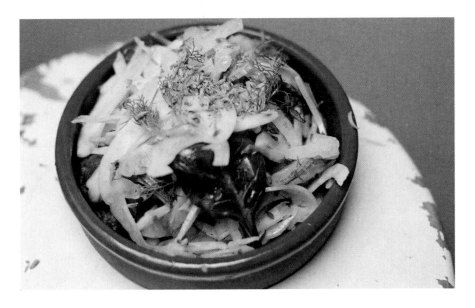

SALAD WITH FENNEL, LEMON & LAVENDER

2 tbsp extra virgin olive oil
zest and juice of 1 lemon
2 tbsp dried lavender flowers
3 fennel bulbs, grated into thin slices, preferably using a mandoline (see page 173)
handful of baby leaf spinach
salt and freshly ground black pepper
gomashio, to serve (see page 75)

Serves 2–4

In a bowl, mix together the olive oil, lemon juice and zest and lavender. Add the fennel and stir to combine. Leave to marinate for 30 minutes, then add the spinach.

Season with salt and pepper and spoon the gomashio on top, to serve.

Lavender contains the well-known phytochemical limonene, which is said to stimulate the detoxification of the liver.

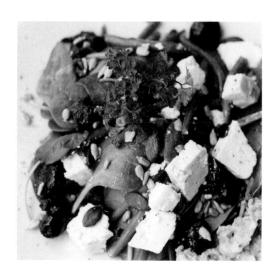

FRESH SUMMER SALAD WITH FETA & BASIL

20g (⅔oz) sunflower seeds
2 large handfuls of seasonal lettuce leaves
50g (1¾oz) sun-dried tomatoes, cut into pieces
1 avocado
150g (5oz) feta cheese
50g (1¾oz) olives (whichever type you prefer)
2 tbsp extra virgin olive oil
1 tbsp apple cider vinegar
salt and freshly ground black pepper
fresh basil leaves (to garnish)

Serves 2

First, toast the sunflower seeds. Set a frying pan over a gentle heat, add the seeds and cook, stirring occasionally, until golden.

Put the lettuce and tomatoes into a serving dish. Cut the avocado flesh into cubes and add to the dish (alternatively, you can roughly mash the avocado and serve on the side). Cut the feta cheese into small cubes, or crush with your hands, and add to the salad along with the olives, then drizzle over the olive oil and cider vinegar. Season with salt and pepper.

Garnish with the toasted sunflower seeds and basil leaves, and serve. If basil is out of season, you can use parsley instead.

This salad is best eaten immediately, but if you need to prepare it in advance, don't add the avocado until serving, and drizzle with lemon juice to prevent it going brown.

Coriander seeds and leaves have traditionally been used to stimulate digestion in both Chinese and Ayurvedic medicine. They're often combined with caraway, cardamom, fennel or anise seeds.

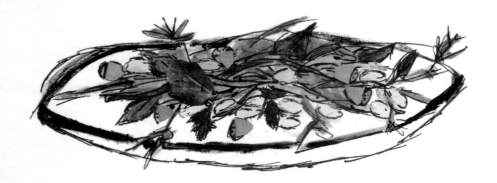

GREEN SPRING SALAD WITH COURGETTE & KUMQUAT

juice of 1 lemon

2 tbsp extra virgin olive oil

2 courgettes, sliced into 'spaghetti' using a mandoline, or grated

100g (3½oz) baby leaf spinach

1 bunch fresh parsley, chopped

7–9 kumquats, halved (if they're not in season or difficult to find, you can use an orange, peeled and cut into small pieces)

25g (⅞oz) sunflower seeds

100g (3½oz) white beans, cooked according to the packet instructions

1 tsp coriander seeds, ground

salt and freshly ground black pepper

Serves 2–4

Put all the ingredients in a bowl, mix well and serve as a side salad or main meal.

RED AUTUMN SALAD

1 small celeriac, peeled
300g (11oz) beetroot, peeled
1 pomegranate (if in season), deseeded (see right)
1 bunch radishes, thinly sliced (you can reserve the
leaves to use as a garnish)
3 tbsp extra virgin olive oil
1 tbsp cider vinegar

Serves 2–4

Grate the celeriac and beetroot, starting with the celeriac, as the red colour
of the beets can easily get everywhere.

Mix all the ingredients together.

Serve with some seeds sprinkled on top, or just a few radish leaves.

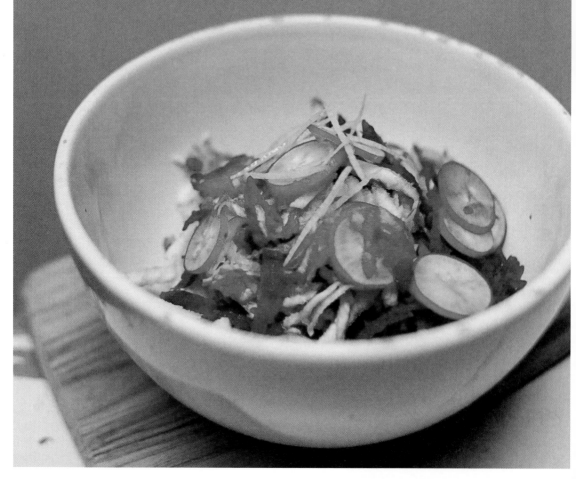

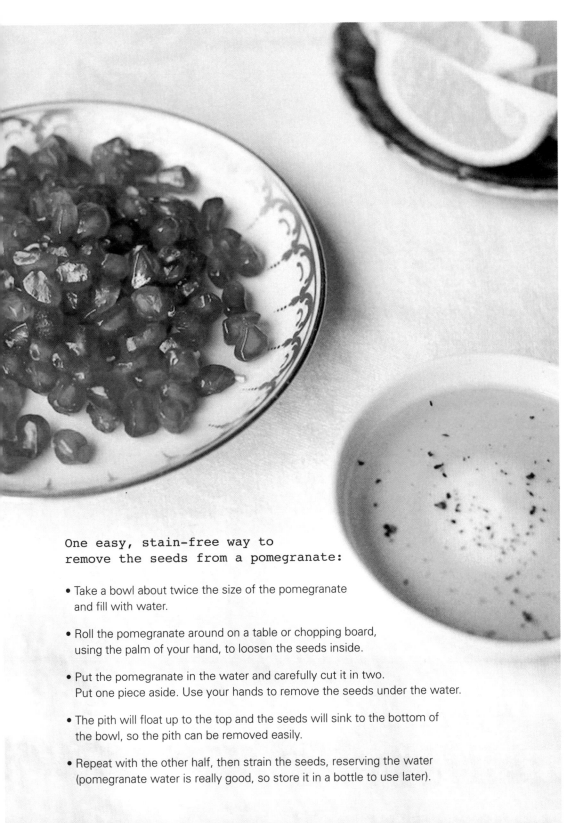

One easy, stain-free way to
remove the seeds from a pomegranate:

- Take a bowl about twice the size of the pomegranate
  and fill with water.

- Roll the pomegranate around on a table or chopping board,
  using the palm of your hand, to loosen the seeds inside.

- Put the pomegranate in the water and carefully cut it in two.
  Put one piece aside. Use your hands to remove the seeds under the water.

- The pith will float up to the top and the seeds will sink to the bottom of
  the bowl, so the pith can be removed easily.

- Repeat with the other half, then strain the seeds, reserving the water
  (pomegranate water is really good, so store it in a bottle to use later).

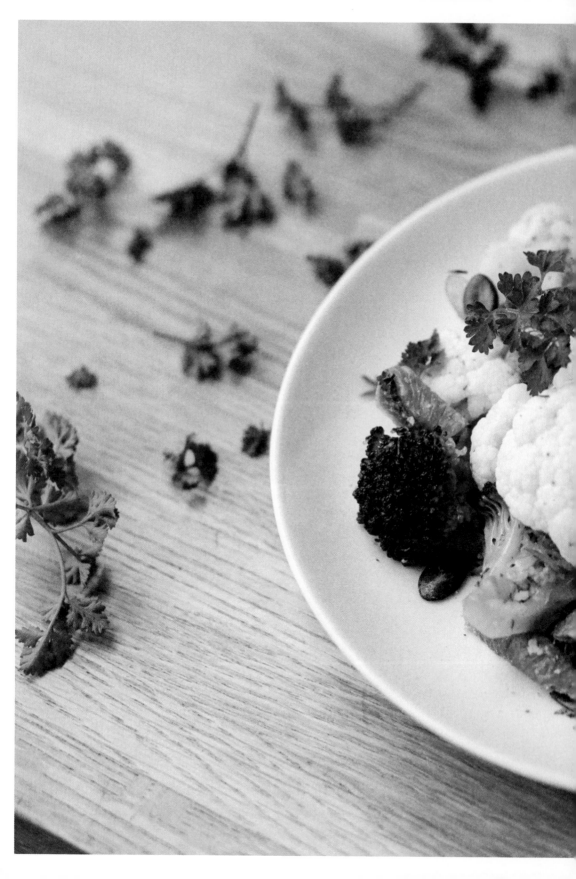

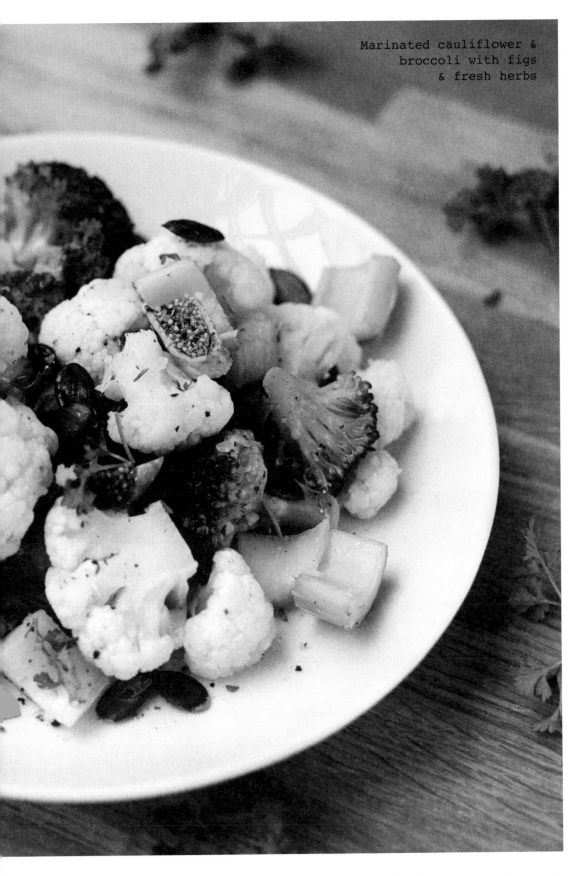

MARINATED CAULIFLOWER & BROCCOLI WITH FIGS & FRESH HERBS

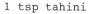

4 tbsp extra virgin olive oil
zest and juice of 1–2 lemons
1 tsp tahini
½ tsp ground cumin
1cm (⅓in) piece fresh root ginger, grated
1 cauliflower, trimmed and cut into florets
1 head of broccoli, trimmed and cut into florets
20g (⅔oz) pumpkin seeds
1 bunch fresh parsley
2 sticks of celery, cut into small pieces
3 fresh figs (if in season; otherwise, use dried),
cut into small pieces
salt and freshly ground black pepper

Serves 2–4 (depending on the size of the cauliflower and whether the dish is served as a side or main)

Put the olive oil, lemon zest and juice, tahini, cumin and ginger in a bowl and mix well with a spoon. Add the cauliflower and broccoli and mix with your hands, to make sure all the florets are coated with the dressing. Leave to marinate in a bowl or bag, preferably for a few hours.

Preheat the oven to 150°C/300°F/Gas 2.

Spread out the pumpkin seeds on a baking sheet and toast in the oven for 10 minutes. Leave to cool.

Add the pumpkin seeds, parsley, celery and figs to the salad, season to taste and serve.

Broccoli is very rich in vitamin C and magnesium, and has many great health benefits.

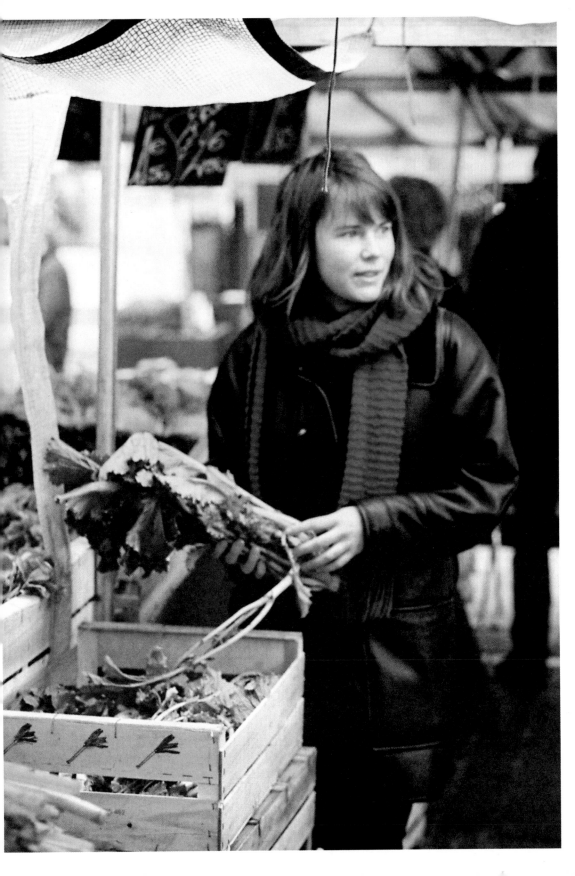

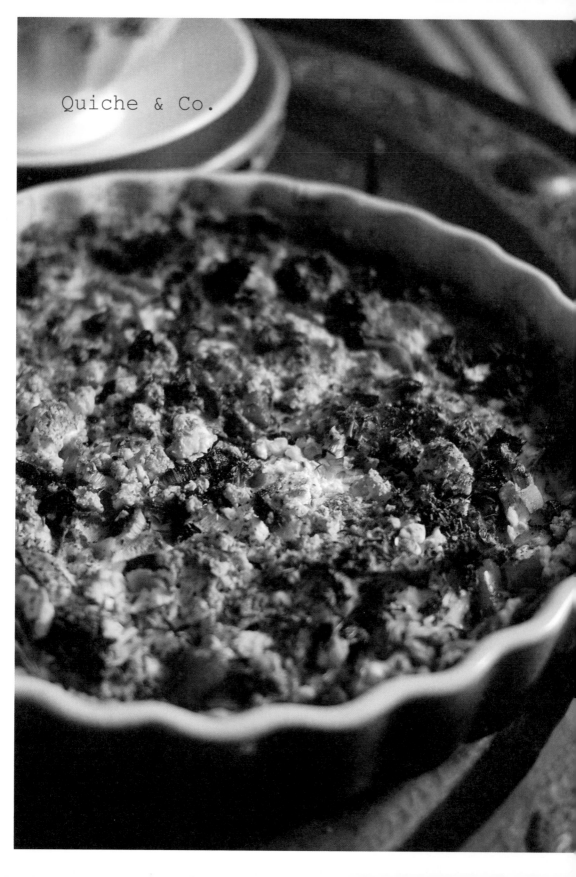

Quiche & Co.

GLUTEN-FREE VEGGIE QUICHE

Crust:
90g (3¼oz) quinoa flour
90g (3¼oz) rice flour
90ml (3floz) extra virgin olive oil
1 egg yolk (vegan option: 1 tbsp baking soda mixed with 1 tbsp white vinegar)
2 tbsp water

Filling:
2 eggs (vegan option: 2 tbsp flaxseeds, 6 tbsp water, 1 tbsp tahini or almond butter, 1 tbsp fibre husk, well mixed)
200g (7oz) oat milk
salt and freshly ground black pepper
1 small courgette, cut into semi-circles
½ broccoli head, cut into small florets
1 red pepper, deseeded and chopped
½ leek, thinly sliced
1 tbsp fresh herbs, chopped (oregano, basil, thyme, rosemary — use any combination you like)
30g (1oz) pitted black olives, halved
70g (2¼oz) feta cheese, cut into cubes or crumbled in your hands (optional)

This veggie quiche contains a good amount of protein and is ideal for including in your lunch box with some fresh salad. Try different combinations of vegetables, to keep it varied!

Serves 3–4

You will need a tart tin 22cm (8½in) in diameter and 2.5cm (1in) deep.

Start by preparing the crust. Mix the flours together in a bowl, then stir in the wet ingredients until well combined. Use your hands to press the dough into the tart tin, then place in the fridge to cool for 2–4 hours.

Preheat the oven to 200°C/400°F/Gas 6. Put the eggs, milk and seasoning in a jug and whisk to combine.

Remove the tart tin from the fridge and put it in the oven for 10 minutes, to blind-bake the crust. Take the crust out of the oven and add the vegetables, herbs, olives and feta cheese (reserve a handful to sprinkle on the top). Pour in the egg mixture, covering the other ingredients, then sprinkle the remaining cheese on top.

Bake in the middle of the oven for 50–60 minutes, until set.

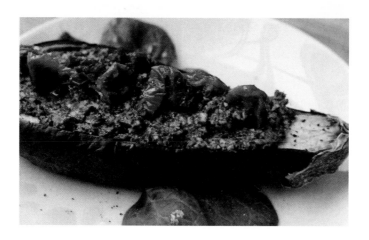

BAKED AUBERGINE WITH GREEN-LEAF PESTO

1 aubergine, halved lengthways
extra virgin olive oil or coconut oil
salt and freshly ground black pepper

Topping:
green-leaf pesto (see page 64)
sun-dried tomatoes

Serves 1–2

Preheat the oven to 180°C/350°F/Gas 4.

Take the aubergine halves and, with a knife, score lines in the flesh in both
directions, to create small squares. Put the two pieces on a baking sheet, pour
some oil over the top and, using your hands, massage the oil in well to make sure
it's really absorbed. Sprinkle on some salt and pepper and bake in the middle of
the oven for about 30 minutes, or until the aubergine is cooked.

Serve with some green-leaf pesto and sun-dried tomatoes on top. This is great as
a side or a starter, and can be adapted to make tasty canapés: when the aubergines
come out of the oven, cut them into 1cm (⅓in) slices, top with the pesto and some
fresh herbs, then put a cocktail stick in each piece and serve to your guests!

Another idea to try:
After 30 minutes, take the aubergine out of the oven and add some tomato
purée and goat's cheese, then bake for another 7 minutes. Then add the pesto
and sun-dried tomatoes.

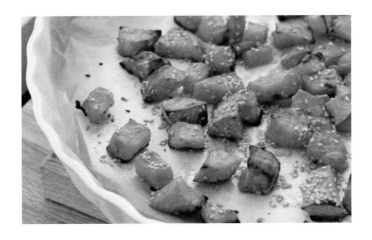

BAKED SWEET POTATO WITH LEMON ZEST & SESAME SEEDS

1 medium-sized sweet potato, cut into small cubes
1 tbsp extra virgin coconut oil
pinch of salt
1 pinch cayenne pepper
2 tsp sesame seeds
zest of 1 lemon

Serves 2

Preheat the oven to 175°C/350°F/Gas 4.

Put the sweet potato cubes in an ovenproof dish and add the coconut oil, spreading it all over the cubes (if the oil is hard, you can use your hands to massage it into the potato; the oil will melt straight away, because of the heat from your hands).

Sprinkle the salt and cayenne pepper over the sweet potatoes, followed by the sesame seeds. Put the dish in the oven and bake for 30–40 minutes, until the potatoes are baked.

Sprinkle the lemon zest over the sweet potatoes.

You can serve this dish hot or cold with your favourite vegetables. Why not try it with seaweed, for a fresh and nourishing salad?

Sweet potatoes are rich in beta-carotene, an antioxidant that helps protect against cell damage and also supports the immune system.

VEGGIE PIZZA

Dough:
90g (3¼oz) extra virgin olive oil
120g (4¼oz) buckwheat flour
120g (4¼oz) cornflour
60g (2oz) rice flour
300ml (½ pint) hot water
¾ tsp salt
any herbs and spices of your choice

Tomato sauce:
60g (2oz) tomato purée
1 tbsp chopped fresh basil
1 tbsp chopped fresh oregano
salt and freshly ground black pepper

Topping:
1 red pepper, deseeded and chopped
½ leek, thinly sliced
½ aubergine, chopped
½ courgette, chopped
25g (⅛oz) pitted black olives, halved
70g (2¼oz) feta cheese, cut into cubes

Serves 2–4

Preheat the oven to 200°C/400°F/Gas 6.

First, prepare the dough. In a bowl, combine the oil and 60g (2oz) of the buckwheat flour, then the remaining flours and the hot water. Add the salt and any herbs and spices to the dough.

Knead the dough, then form it into a pizza shape and transfer to a baking sheet. Use your hands to press out the dough and form an edge around the outside. Bake for 10 minutes.

Meanwhile, prepare the tomato sauce. Put the tomato purée, herbs and seasoning into a small saucepan over a low heat and bring to the boil, stirring continuously. Spread over the baked pizza dough, then top with the vegetables, olives and feta cheese. Bake in the middle of the oven for 35 minutes.

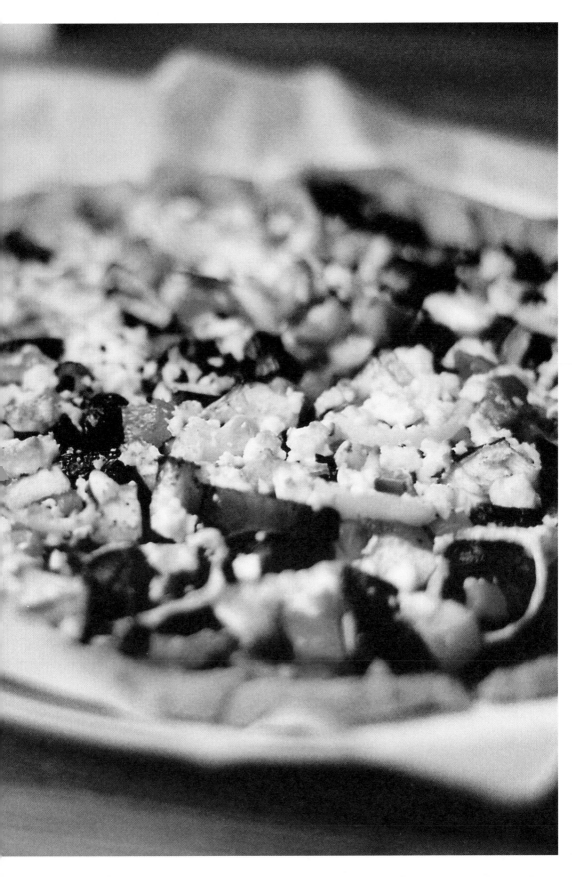

I used to work in a quality food store in Stockholm, where I held cooking events, and I sometimes worked with a man who was very well known for his knowledge and experience of making sushi. I would ask him if he could – and should – pioneer sushi made with brown rice. I thought it was a brilliant idea, and I was sure it would be as good as standard sushi, but more filling and more nutritious. In the end, I was the one going home and trying it out, and here is my result …

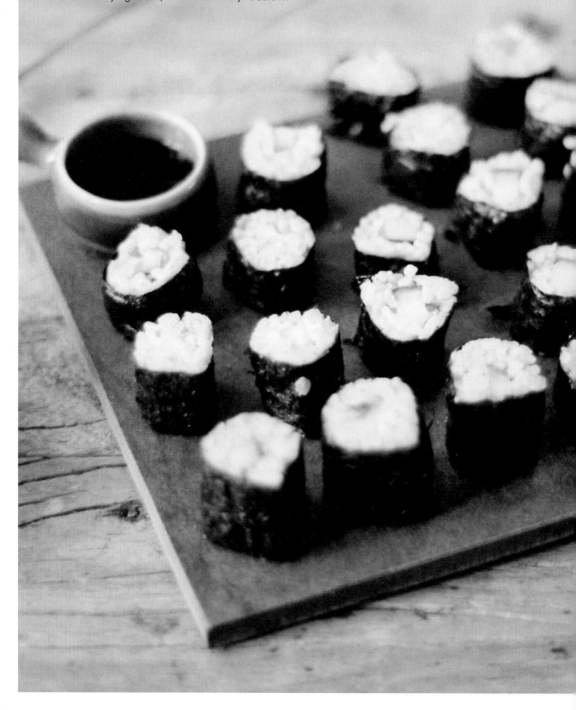

GREEN TAMARI NORI ROLLS

Sticky rice:
150g (5oz) short-grain brown rice

Sauce:
1 tbsp extra virgin olive oil
1½ tbsp lemon juice
salt and freshly ground black pepper
1–2 tsp apple cider vinegar
1 tbsp tahini

4–6 sheets nori
1 avocado, chopped
½ cucumber, cut into long sticks
homemade gomashio (see page 75)
about 2 tbsp tamari soy sauce
2cm (¾ in) piece fresh root ginger,
peeled and grated

Rice boosts the metabolism and promotes healthy hair and skin.

Serves 2–4

Cook the rice according to the packet instructions. Leave to cool naturally or by putting the rice in a bowl and then in ice-cold water.

To prepare the sauce, put the olive oil, lemon juice, salt and pepper, apple cider vinegar and tahini in a bowl and mix well (tilting the bowl as you do so), until it takes on a creamy beige colour. Add the rice to the sauce and combine. The mixture should have a nice creamy, sticky texture; if it isn't sticky enough, you can add some more tahini and lemon juice. Taste the rice and, if you wish, add some spices.

Make sure your work surface is nice and clean, ready to make the rolls. Lay out the first sheet of nori and spread some of the sticky rice in a strip along the bottom. Lay some avocado and cucumber on top of the rice, sprinkle over some gomashio and then roll up the nori tightly. Brush with water so that the roll sticks together.

Slice the roll into thick pieces and repeat the rolling process with the remaining ingredients.

Dip the nori rolls in some tamari and ginger. Enjoy!

You can experiment with different ingredients – instead of cucumber, I often use courgette, carrot or celery.

TORTILLA

4 eggs
salt and freshly ground black pepper
pinch of dried thyme
1 tbsp extra virgin olive oil
½ onion
2 garlic cloves, crushed
1 carrot, scrubbed and grated
1 red pepper, thinly sliced into rings

Serves 2

Crack the eggs into a bowl, add some salt and pepper and the dried thyme, and whisk with a fork.

Heat the olive oil in a frying pan over a medium heat, add the vegetables and fry gently, stirring continuously, for about 4 minutes, until slightly softened and golden. Add the eggs and slowly tilt the pan in all directions, to spread them evenly over the base. Watch the pan to make sure the tortilla doesn't burn.

When the tortilla is nicely cooked underneath and moves freely in the pan, fold it in half and cook for a little longer. Turn it over and cook the other side. You can either leave it a bit soft in the middle or cook it thoroughly all the way through – whichever way you prefer.

Serve with a fresh green salad, some homemade crackers (see pages 54–56) or just as it is.

Soups

GREEN GASPACHO

1 courgette, chopped
½ avocado
½ cucumber, peeled if you wish
(I prefer to leave the skin on),
and chopped
small handful of green kale, chopped
juice of 1 lemon, freshly squeezed
2 tbsp extra virgin olive oil
1 tsp spirulina powder
1 small bunch fresh coriander, chopped
salt and freshly ground black pepper
200ml (7 floz) cold filtered water

Serves 2

Put all the ingredients in a blender (or you can use a hand mixer), adding the water
a little at a time, and whizz until smooth. You may find that your blender can't cut
through the hard stems of the kale, in which case just use the leafy parts. Taste
the gaspacho, adding more lemon juice and seasoning if necessary.

Delicious served with some fresh tomatoes or a sprinkling of nuts and seeds.

*Super-easy and healthy fast food, with a mix of healthy
fats and antioxidants, and loaded with chlorophyll.*

My favourite summer soup!

PARSNIP & COCONUT SOUP

2–3 parsnips (about 400g/14oz), chopped
into medium-sized chunks
3 cloves garlic
extra virgin coconut oil (for roasting)
salt and freshly ground black pepper
1 tsp cumin seeds
½ tsp ground turmeric
1 tsp ground ginger
½ tsp mustard seeds
300ml (11floz) water
400ml (13½floz) can coconut milk
1 tsp sesame oil

Serves 2

Preheat the oven to 180°C/350°F/Gas 4. Place the parsnips on a baking sheet, together with the garlic cloves. Drizzle with coconut oil and season with salt and pepper. Bake for about 45 minutes, until nicely roasted and tender.

Transfer the parsnips and garlic to a large saucepan and add the spices and water. Cook over a low heat, uncovered, for about 10 minutes, stirring occasionally to activate the flavours of the spices and to ensure the parsnips are evenly cooked.

Add the coconut milk and sesame oil, and whizz with a hand blender until smooth. If the soup is too thick, you can add more water. Gently warm the soup through again before serving.

This is my favourite comfort soup, with a blend of anti-inflammatory spices and creamy coconut!

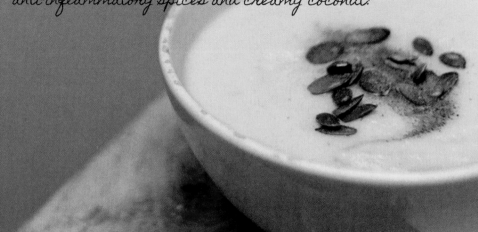

CREAMY SWEET POTATO SOUP WITH COCONUT & CARROT

2 tbsp extra virgin coconut oil
1 onion, chopped
2 carrots, cut into small pieces
1 sweet potato, cut into small cubes
1cm (⅓in) piece fresh root ginger,
peeled and grated
1cm (⅓in) piece fresh turmeric root,
peeled and grated, or 1 tsp ground turmeric
pinch of salt
pinch of freshly ground black pepper
300ml (½ pint) coconut milk

Serves 2

Heat the coconut oil in a saucepan and add the onion, frying gently for about
2 minutes or until golden. Add the carrots and sweet potato and continue to cook
for a few more minutes, stirring from time to time to prevent burning. Stir in the
ginger and turmeric, then add just enough water to cover the vegetables and season
with the salt and pepper. Simmer for 20 minutes, until the vegetables are softened.

Add the coconut milk and bring to the boil, then remove from the heat and whizz
with a hand blender. Taste the soup and adjust the flavours if necessary.

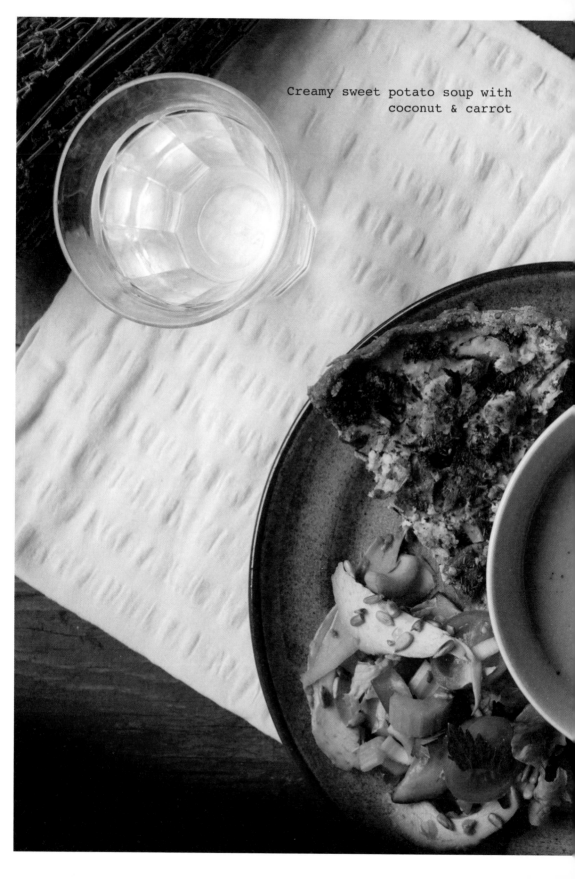

Creamy sweet potato soup with
coconut & carrot

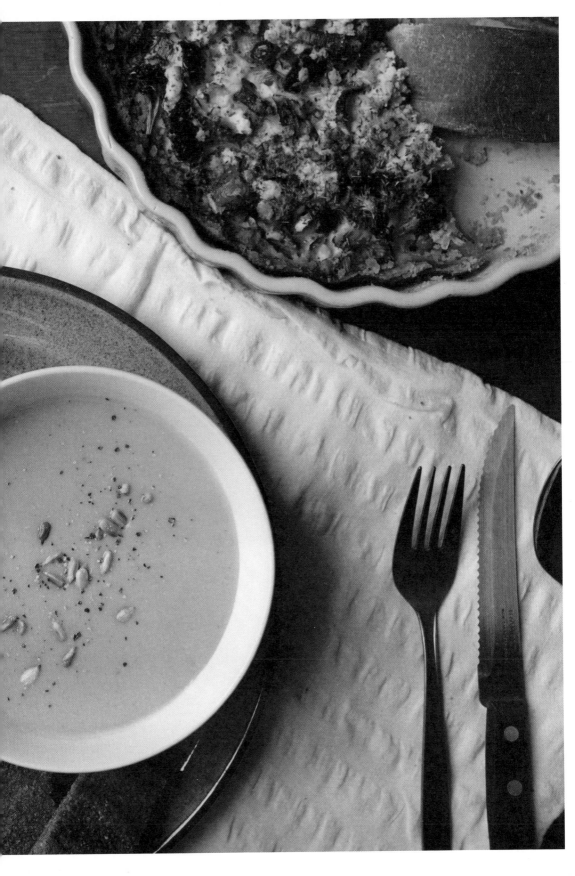

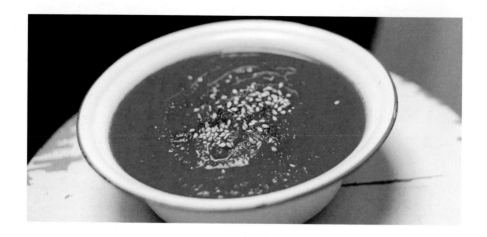

BEETROOT SOUP WITH CUMIN & CARDAMOM

2 tsp extra virgin coconut oil
1 onion, chopped
1 small fennel bulb, chopped
2 garlic cloves, finely chopped
500g (1lb 2oz) beetroot
sea salt
freshly ground black pepper
1 tsp ground cumin
½ tsp ground cardamom
1 tsp lemon zest
800ml (1½ pints) water

Serves 2

Heat the oil in a large saucepan or soup pot, over a medium heat. Add the onion, fennel and garlic and cook, stirring every now and then, for about 10 minutes or until softened.

Add the beets, along with the salt, pepper, spices and lemon zest, then pour in the water to cover the vegetables. Turn the heat up to high and bring the soup to the boil, then cover and leave to simmer for 40–60 minutes, or until the vegetables are soft.

Turn off the heat and carefully whizz with a hand blender. Taste the soup and season with more spices if needed. Add some fresh herbs and a grind of black pepper, or a sprinkling of sesame seeds, and serve with some crackers.

Beetroot is traditionally valued for its detoxifying properties, as it helps to purify the blood and the liver!

BUTTERNUT SQUASH & CARROT SOUP WITH SAFFRON

2 tbsp extra virgin coconut oil

1 onion, chopped

1 butternut squash (weighing about 1 kg/2lb 3oz), peeled and chopped

2 medium-sized carrots, chopped

¼ tsp saffron

2cm (¾in) piece fresh turmeric root, peeled and finely chopped (take care, as it can easily stain your clothes)

salt and freshly ground black pepper

1–1.25 litres (1¾–2¼ pints) water

Serves 2–4

Heat the coconut oil in a large saucepan, then add the onion and cook for 4–6 minutes, stirring regularly, until nicely golden. Add the remaining vegetables, spices and seasoning, and cover with the water. Simmer for 20–30 minutes, until the vegetables are softened.

Whizz the soup with a hand blender, until you have a smooth texture. Let it simmer for a few minutes more, before serving.

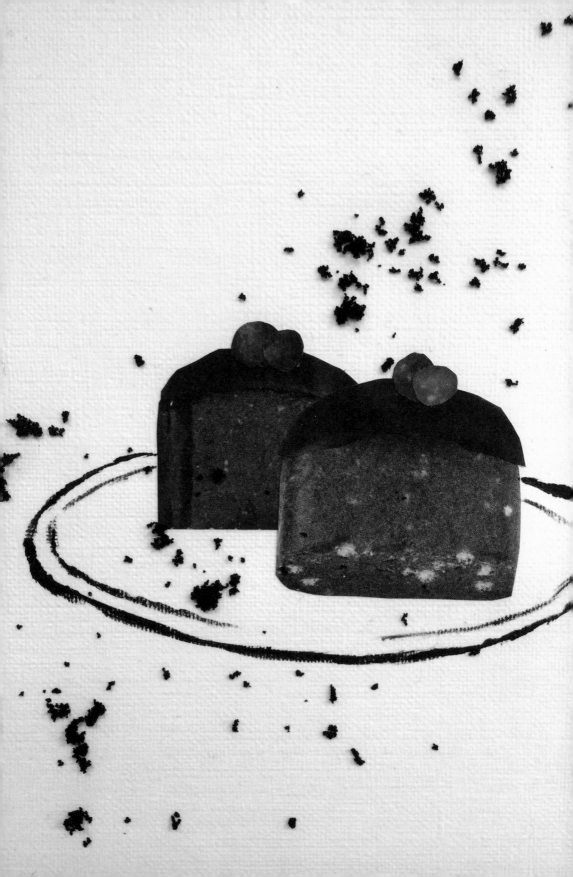

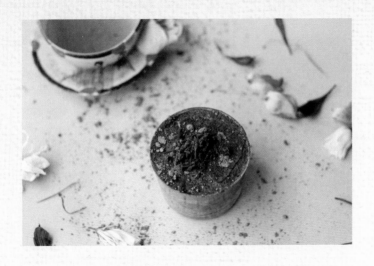

SWEET TREATS

I like to keep my treats simple and use only
natural ingredients; I also like to experiment
to find foods that contain a natural sweetness.
We don't need to add white sugar to our
desserts; there are so many sweet options
that don't give you a massive blood-sugar spike
and energy low, but just give you a sweet,
nutritious treat.

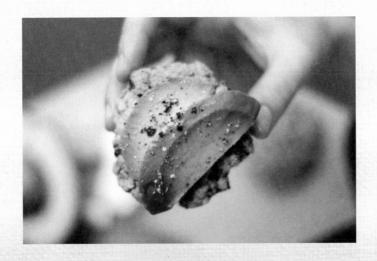

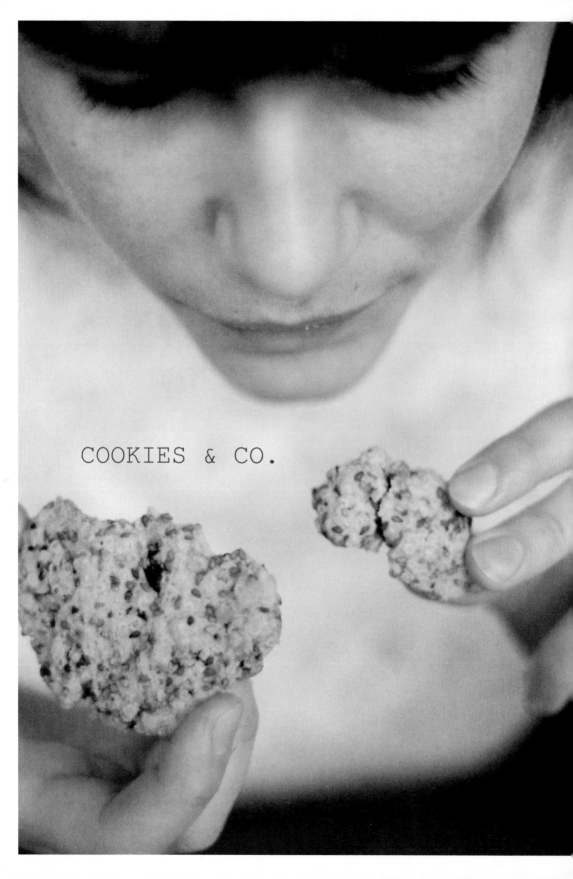

COOKIES & CO.

GRAINY QUINOA COOKIES

100g (3½oz) quinoa flakes
50g (1¾oz) sesame seeds
50g (1¾oz) pumpkin seeds
50g (1¾oz) sunflower seeds
50g (1¾oz) cornflour
50g (1¾oz) almond flour
1 tbsp honey (or agave syrup)
30g (1oz) extra virgin olive oil
2 eggs (vegan option: 1 tbsp flaxseeds,
3 tbsp water and 1 tbsp almond milk)
2 pinches of salt

Makes 10–14 cookies

Preheat the oven to 180°C/350°F/Gas 4 and lightly grease a baking sheet.

Mix all the ingredients together in a bowl, then knead the dough with your hands.

Divide the dough into 10–14 pieces (each one should weigh about 60g/2oz), shape them into balls, then flatten to make thin cookies and place them on a baking sheet.

Bake in the middle of the oven for 8 minutes, then turn the baking sheet and bake for another 8 minutes.

Quinoa is a great source of vegetable protein and helps to build muscle strength!

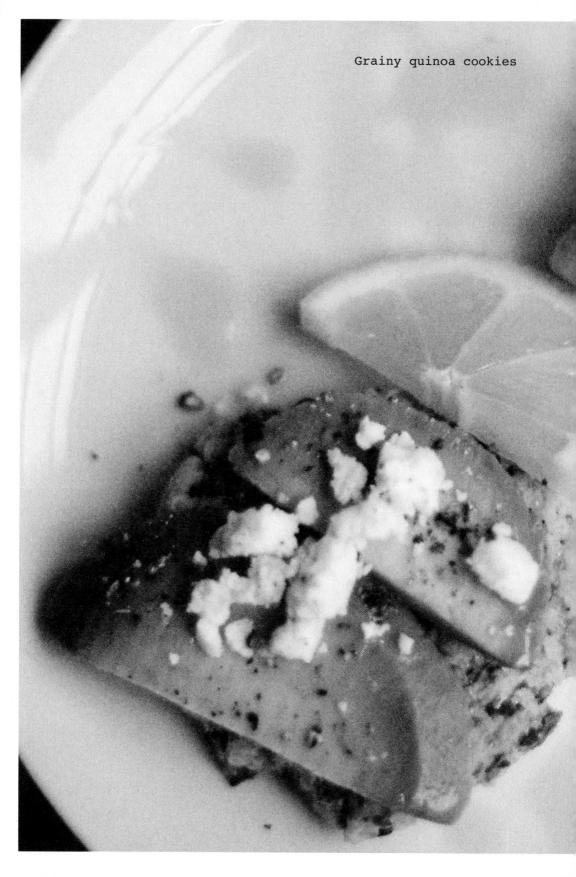

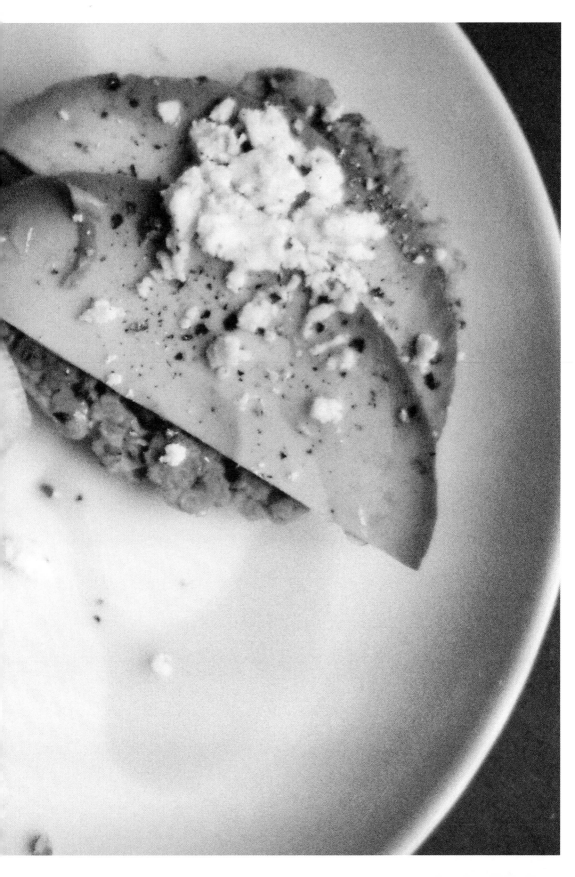

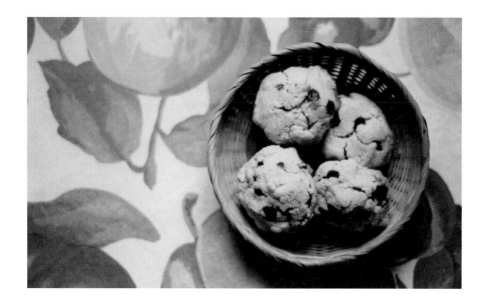

BISCUIT BITES

50g (1¾oz) almond flour
50g (1¾oz) rice flour
1 tsp baking powder
2 tsp chocolate (your favourite chocolate
broken into small pieces)
50ml (2floz) oat milk
2 tsp extra virgin coconut oil
2 tsp honey (or agave syrup)

Makes 4 small biscuits

Preheat the oven to 180°C/350°F/Gas 4 and lightly grease a baking sheet.

Combine the flours, baking powder and chocolate in a bowl, then add the milk,
oil and honey, to form a dough.

Divide the dough into 4 pieces and shape into rounds using your hands, then flatten
slightly (they should still be fairly rounded). Place them on the baking sheet on the
middle oven shelf and bake for 16 minutes.

SAVOURY CARROT SCONES

35g (1¼oz) flaxseeds
50ml (2floz) hot water
2 small carrots (about 125g/4½oz), grated
40g (1½oz) pumpkin seeds
100g (3½oz) buckwheat flakes
40g (1½oz) sunflower seeds
1 tsp baking powder
1½ tbsp extra virgin olive oil
1 tsp salt

Makes 6 scones

Soak the flaxseeds in the hot water for at least 1 hour.

Preheat the oven to 175°C/350°F/Gas 4 and lightly grease a baking sheet.

Put the carrots in a bowl with the soaked flaxseeds. Add the remaining ingredients and mix everything together. Don't worry if the texture feels dry; the moisture from the carrot will gradually be released into the dough.

Knead the dough thoroughly, then divide into 6 pieces and form into rounds. Each scone should weigh about 60g (2oz). Place them on the baking sheet and bake in the middle of the oven for 25–35 minutes.

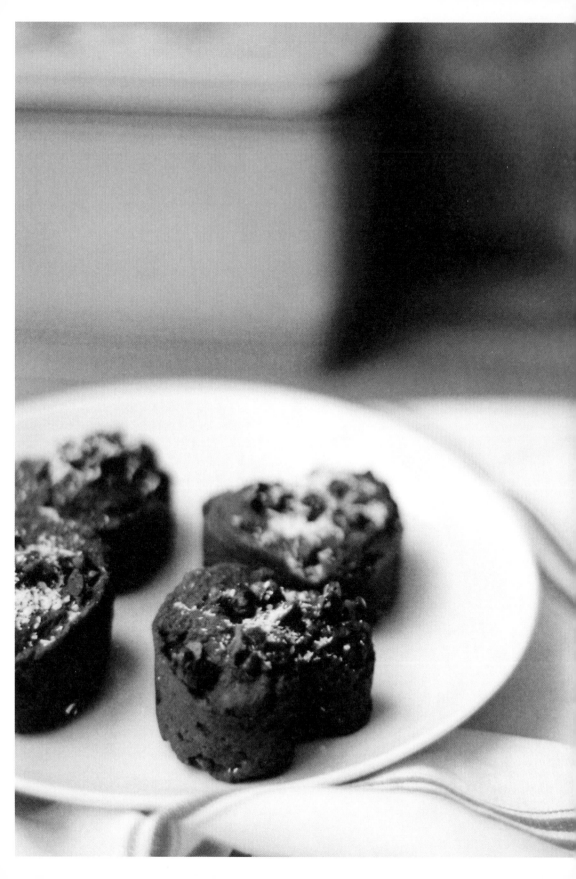

CHOCO CHILLI MUFFINS

2 bananas, mashed
2 tbsp extra virgin coconut oil
2 eggs (vegan option: 1 tbsp flaxseeds,
3 tbsp water and 1 tbsp almond milk)
3 tbsp cacao powder
1 tbsp honey (or agave syrup)
1 tsp baking powder
pinch of salt
100g (3½oz) almond flour
25g (⅞oz) coconut flour
60g (2oz) rice flour
pinch of chilli powder (optional)
coconut flakes or chocolate pieces, to sprinkle
on top (optional)

Makes 6–8 muffins

Line a muffin tin with small muffin cups (about 4cm/1½in in diameter). Preheat the oven to 180°C/350°F/Gas 4.

Put the bananas and coconut oil in a large mixing bowl and mix together to form a creamy texture. Stir in the eggs, cacao powder and honey, then add the baking powder and salt, and combine. Last of all, add the flours and chilli powder, then mix thoroughly with a fork, until all the ingredients are well incorporated.

Spoon the batter into the muffin cups (each muffin should weigh about 60g/2oz). The texture of these muffins is pretty compact, so don't worry if the batter seems quite dry – this is normal.

Sprinkle over the coconut flakes or chocolate pieces (if using), and bake in the middle of the oven for 20 minutes.

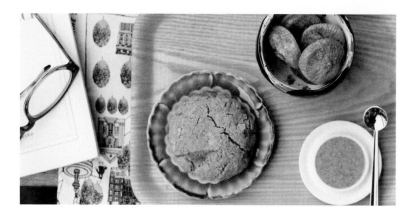

ALMOND & FIG SCONES

4 dried figs, cut into small pieces (preferably soaked
in water for a minimum of 1 hour)

150ml (5 fl oz) hot water

100g (3½ oz) almond flour

200g (7oz) crushed or flaked almonds

300g (11oz) buckwheat flour

2 tsp baking powder

1 tsp salt

1 tsp honey
(or agave syrup)

Buckwheat is a gluten-free grain high in protein and fibre – gentle on the stomach and easy to digest.

Makes 6 large round scones

Soaking the figs will make them more moist, but if you don't have the time or
forget to do it, don't worry – just use them as they are.

Preheat the oven to 200°C/400°F/Gas 4 and lightly grease a baking sheet.

Put the water on to boil while you mix all the dry ingredients together in a bowl.
Now add some of the water (don't add it all at once – you may not need it all), along
with the honey and the figs, and – with your hands or a spoon – knead into a dough.
The texture of the dough should be pretty sticky; you don't want it to be too wet or
too dry, so add as much of the remaining water as required.

Divide the dough into 6 pieces, form into round scones and place on the baking
sheet. Bake in the middle of the oven for 12 minutes.

Enjoy warm, fresh from the oven …

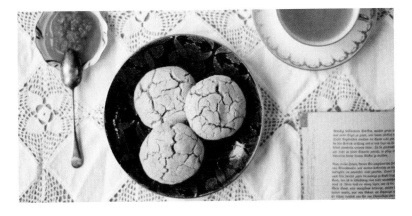

PLAIN SCONES

This is a very basic scone recipe – I want to give you a good base with which to play around and make your own versions, using different flavours. You can use any types of flour and milk.

180g (6¼oz) rice flour
120g (4¼oz) buckwheat flour
1–2 tsp honey (optional)
150–200ml (5–7floz) rice milk
2 tsp baking powder
1 tsp salt

Makes about 6 scones

Preheat the oven to 200°C/400°F/Gas 6 and lightly grease a baking sheet.

Combine all the ingredients in a mixing bowl, starting with 150ml (5fl oz) milk, adding more if needed (the dough needs to be stiff enough to form into balls).

With floured hands, divide the dough into 6 pieces and roll into balls. The dough might be a bit sticky, depending on what flours you're using; this is normal, and is a good sign, as it should mean that your scones won't be dry.

Flatten the balls a little, place on the baking sheet, and bake in the middle of the oven for 12 minutes. Remove from the oven and enjoy warm.

CHOCOLATE COOKIES

90g (3¼oz) buckwheat flour
60g (2oz) cornflour
25g (⅞oz) almond flour
2 tsp baking powder
1 tbsp cacao powder
pinch of salt
2 eggs (vegan option: 1 tbsp flaxseeds,
3 tbsp water and 1 tbsp almond milk)
2 tbsp honey or maple syrup
90g (3¼oz) butter (or dairy free: 45g coconut oil
and 45g olive oil)
35g (1¼oz) dark chocolate chips

Makes 6–8 cookies

Preheat the oven to 180°C/350°F/Gas 4 and line a baking sheet with baking parchment.

Put the flours in a bowl, add the baking powder, cacao powder and salt, and mix all the dry ingredients together. Now add the eggs, honey, butter/oils and chocolate chips, and mix thoroughly until the dough has a creamy texture.

To make the cookies, divide the dough into 6–8 balls and then flatten these with your hands to form rounds about 1cm (⅓in) thick (if the dough is very sticky, dust your hands with some cacao powder or flour before forming the cookie shapes).

Place the cookies on the lined baking sheet and bake in the middle of the oven for around 15 minutes. They should still be a bit soft in the middle when ready, so, depending on your oven, you might need to take them out a couple of minutes earlier.

Delicious served with a little almond butter.

A sweet snack-time treat containing a good amount of protein to give you that extra bit of energy!

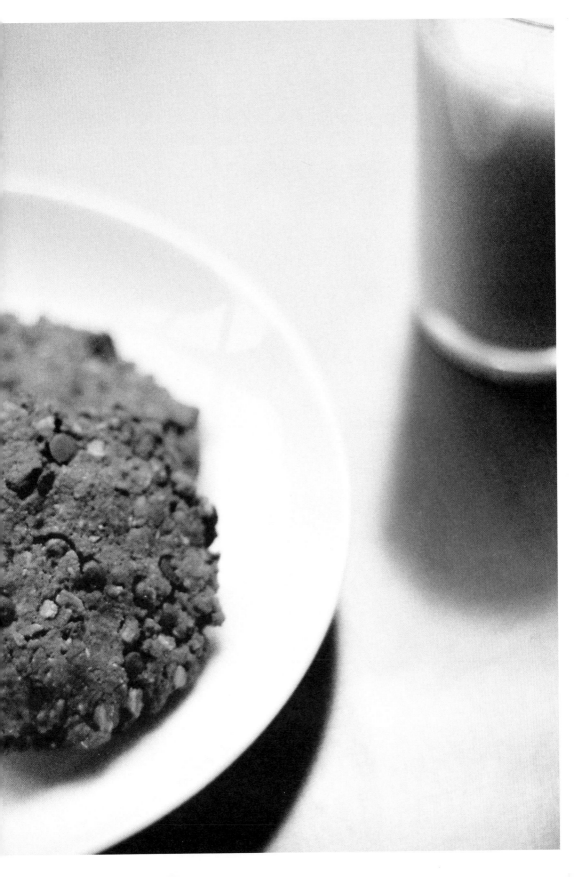

These biscuits are packed with healthy omegas and protein. The cardamom gives a delicious taste and also has many health properties, like helping the digestion and giving that extra energy boost!

CARDAMOM BISCUITS

200g (7oz) raw buckwheat groats
500ml (17floz) water
75g (2½oz) pumpkin seeds
65g (2¼oz) almonds
1 tsp ground cardamom
1 tbsp honey (or agave syrup)
½ tsp ground vanilla
1 tbsp extra virgin coconut oil

Makes about 15 biscuits

Soak the buckwheat groats in the water for at least 30 minutes.

Preheat the oven to 200°C/400°F/Gas 6. Line a baking sheet with baking parchment.

Rinse the buckwheat groats, then put all the ingredients in a food processor and blend to a coarse texture.

Remove the dough and form into a cylinder, then cut into slices about 1cm (⅓in) thick (alternatively, you can form the dough into balls and flatten with your hands).

Place the slices on the baking sheet and bake in the middle of the oven for 11–15 minutes (until cooked, but not burnt!).

This recipe can also be eaten raw – just skip the baking part!

BUCKWHEAT & RICE SCONES WITH SUNFLOWER SEEDS

100g (3½oz) buckwheat flour
100g (3½oz) whole rice flour
75g (2½oz) sunflower seeds
2 tbsp extra virgin coconut oil
2 tsp baking powder
pinch of salt
150ml (5floz) of your preferred milk
(I use almond milk)
dried apricots or figs, cut into pieces (optional)

Makes 5–7 scones

Preheat the oven to 220°C/425°F/Gas 7 and lightly grease a baking sheet.

Combine all the ingredients together in a bowl. If it's winter and the air is cold, your coconut oil will probably be solid, in which case gently heat it in a saucepan, or put it in the oven briefly, so it's melted before you add it to the mixture.

Knead the dough, coating your hands in flour if the dough is very sticky. Divide into pieces and shape into round scones (the number of scones you'll get depends on how large or small you want them). Place them on the baking sheet.

Bake for 10–12 minutes in the middle of the oven, until the scones are cooked and golden in colour.

Serve with your favourite nut butter, jam or other spread of your choice.

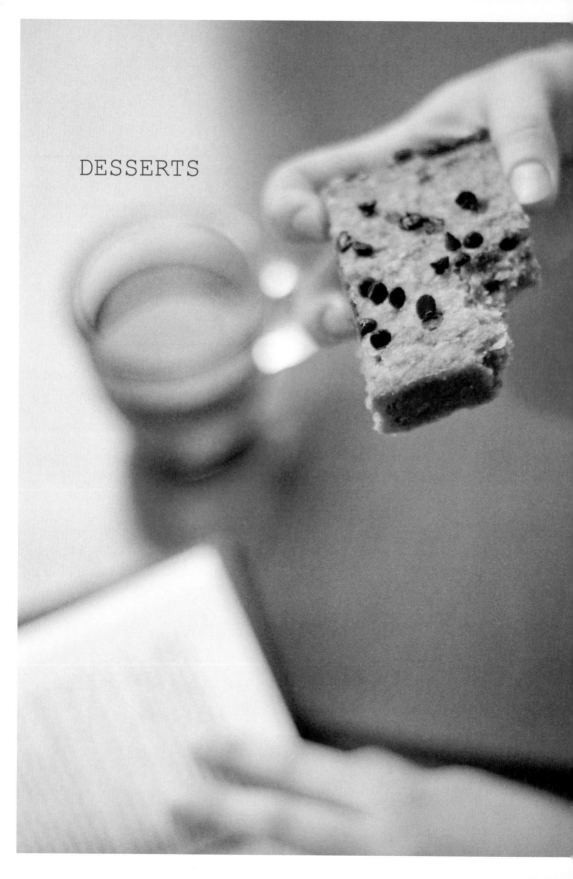

DESSERTS

BANANA BREAD

1 tbsp extra virgin coconut oil, plus extra for greasing

3 bananas, mashed

1 egg (vegan option: 1 tbsp flaxseeds and 3 tbsp vegetable milk — I like to mix one spoon of almond milk with two spoons of rice milk)

1 tsp ground vanilla

1 tsp ground cinnamon

1 tbsp honey or maple syrup

1 tsp baking powder

pinch of salt

150g (5oz) almond flour

30g (1oz) buckwheat flour

35g (1¼oz) coconut flakes

1 tbsp chocolate pieces (made with 100% cacao)

Makes 1 loaf

Preheat the oven to 175°C/350°F/Gas 4. Grease a 900g (2lb) loaf tin with coconut oil.

Put the mashed bananas and coconut oil into a large mixing bowl and mix with a fork until they take on a creamy texture. Stir in the egg, vanilla, cinnamon and your choice of honey or maple syrup. Sprinkle the baking powder and salt over the mixture and combine. Last of all, add the flours and mix.

Sprinkle the coconut flakes over the base and sides of the loaf tin, then pour in the banana mixture. Scatter the chocolate pieces on top and bake in the middle of the oven for 40 minutes.

QUICK APPLE CRUMBLE

45ml (1½floz) extra virgin coconut oil
400g (14oz) apples, cut into small cubes
70g (2¼oz) oat flakes
25g (⅛oz) almond flour
1 tsp ground cinnamon
2 tbsp honey (or agave syrup)
15g (½oz) coconut flakes

Serves 4

Preheat the oven to 220°C/425°F/Gas 7. Grease a 30cm (12in) tart tin with some of the coconut oil.

Put the apples in the tart tin, then cover with the oats, flour and cinnamon, stirring them around with a spoon or your hands to distribute evenly. Stir through the rest of the coconut oil, drizzle the honey over the top, then sprinkle with the coconut flakes.

Bake in the middle of the oven for 20–30 minutes.

Leave to cool before serving. Delicious with vanilla ice cream!

BASIC TART OR PIE

This is a basic pastry recipe for a versatile tart case that you can use for all kinds of sweet or savoury bake.

1 egg (vegan option: 1 tbsp flaxseeds and
3 tbsp almond milk)
150g (5oz) sunflower seeds
50g (1¾oz) pumpkin seeds
1 tbsp chia
50g (1¾oz) quinoa flour
1 tbsp extra virgin olive oil
pinch of salt

Serves 4

Preheat the oven to 175°C/350°F/Gas 4. Grease a 30cm (12in) tart tin.

Crack the egg into a bowl and whisk until quite fluffy, but not white. Add the remaining ingredients and mix to form a dough.

Place the dough in the tart tin and, using your hands, flatten it out until it covers the base and sides of the tin.

Now add your chosen savoury or sweet filling (see suggestion below) and bake in the middle of the oven for 25 minutes.

To make an apple pie, you could add:
2 large apples, cut into small cubes
½ tsp vanilla extract
1 tsp ground cinnamon
2 tbsp honey (or agave syrup)

RAW COCONUT TART WITH CHOCOLATE MOUSSE

Crust:
100g (3½oz) almonds
2 medjool dates
2 tbsp coconut oil
1 pinch bourbon vanilla powder, or the seeds
from half a vanilla pod
1—2 tbsp water

Chocolate mousse:
2 avocados
3 tbsp cacao powder
a little water
pinch of salt
1 tbsp maple syrup or honey (optional)

Serves 4

Start by preparing the crust for the tart. Blend all the ingredients in a food processor until you get a sticky dough (add a little more water if the dough is dry). The texture should feel creamy and moist, so that it can be easily kneaded to create a firm and even base for your tart.

Divide the dough into 4 (if serving individual portions) and press it down into the bottom of your chosen glasses; if serving as a whole tart, then use a tart tin or just press the dough onto a plate. Although the dough is sticky, you'll get the best results if you use your hands to form a nice thin layer, but you can also use a spatula, if you prefer. Leave it in the fridge to harden for around 30 minutes.

Now put all the mousse ingredients (bar the maple syrup/honey) into a clean food processor and blend until really creamy and smooth. The more water you add, the fluffier the mousse gets – but don't add too much! Start with a small spoon of water, and see how you get on; the texture should be fairly heavy, but you're looking for something lighter than a guacamole. Sweeten to taste with the maple syrup/honey, if desired (start by adding a teaspoon, and continue as required).

Check that the crust has hardened, then spread the chocolate mousse on top, using a spatula or spoon. Put your tart(s) back in the fridge again to cool, before serving.

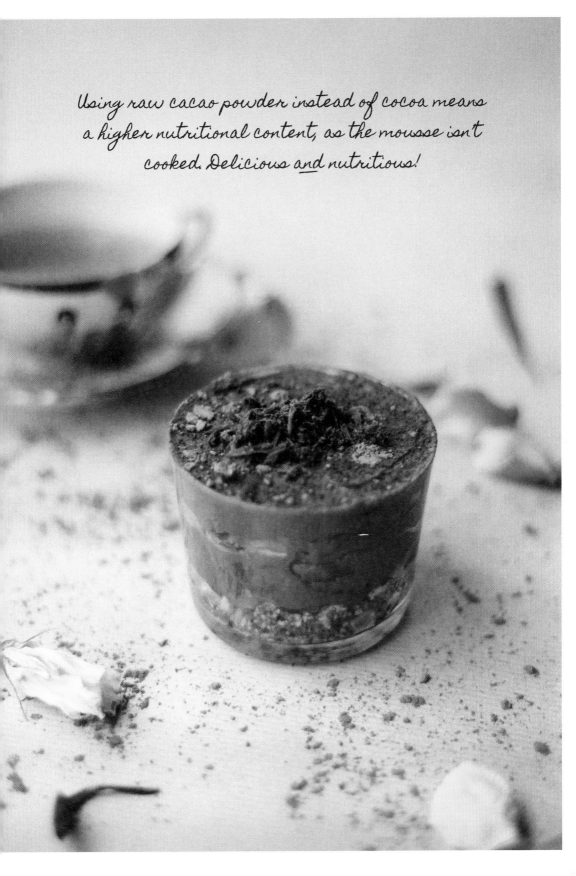

Using raw cacao powder instead of cocoa means a higher nutritional content, as the mousse isn't cooked. Delicious _and_ nutritious!

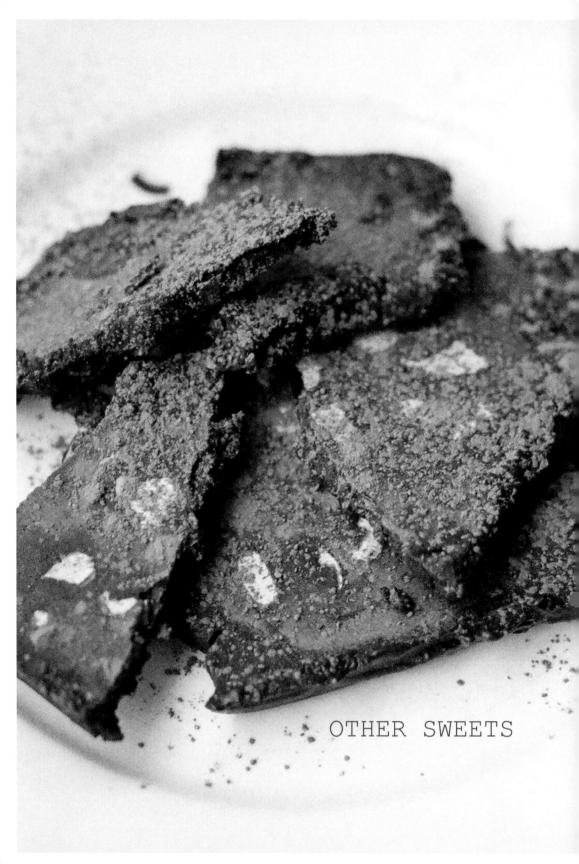

OTHER SWEETS

LINA'S CHOCOLATE

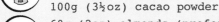

100g (3½oz) raw cacao butter
45g (1½oz) honey (or agave syrup)
100g (3½oz) cacao powder
60g (2oz) almonds (preferably toasted), chopped
pinch of salt
1 tsp ground vanilla
any spices of your choice, such as cayenne pepper,
cardamom, cinnamon …

Makes 8–10 chocolate pieces

You will need a rectangular glass tray or shallow dish, 15 x 10cm (6 x 4 in),
or 8–10 individual moulds (I use an ice cube tray).

Melt the cacao butter in a bowl set over boiling water. Add the honey and stir
until melted and well mixed with the cacao butter.

Combine the rest of the ingredients in a bowl, then add the cacao butter and
honey and stir until the mixture has a very creamy texture.

Pour the chocolate into the dish or mould (each piece should weigh about
20g/⅔ oz), then leave to cool in the fridge for at least 4 hours, before serving.

*My own favourite chocolate, sweetened with honey!
Experiment with other shapes and try different
spices and nuts. A delicious after-dinner treat and
a great gift for a loved one.*

Bananas are rich in potassium, which is essential for controlling the heart rate and blood pressure!

BANANA CHOCO LOLLIPOPS

```
100g (3½oz) chocolate, made with 100% cacao
(or make your own; see Lina's chocolate, page 133)
1 tbsp coconut flakes
2 bananas, cut in half
4 wooden lolly sticks
```

Serves 4

Break the chocolate into pieces and put in a bowl. Heat a saucepan of water over a gentle heat and set the bowl over the water, making sure the water doesn't touch the chocolate. (If you're making Lina's chocolate to use in this recipe, just skip the setting and cooling stage.)

Line a container or plate with baking parchment and put the coconut flakes on a plate. Put a lolly stick into each banana piece and dip them in the melted chocolate and then the coconut flakes. As the chocolate is liquid, you might find it difficult to dip it in the coconut, in which case you can just sprinkle the coconut over the banana using your hands.

Place the bananas in the lined container or on the plate, and leave to cool for at least 3 hours, until the chocolate has set.

CHIA PARFAIT

Perfect 3pm lifesaver – without coffee!

½ banana
2 tbsp chia
1½ tbsp raw cacao
2 tsp maca powder (or other protein powder
or superfood such as hemp protein, mesquite, lucuma …)
pinch of ground vanilla
pinch of ground cinnamon
100ml (3½floz) filtered water

Serves 1–2

Whizz all the ingredients using a blender or hand mixer, and enjoy!

The longer you leave it, the thicker it will become. So, if you want more of
a pudding texture, leave your chia parfait for 20–30 minutes.

*Chia seeds are high in protein, omega-3s
and dietary fibre. This is the perfect
sweet treat, giving you high-quality nutrition!*

COCO CHOCOLATE DREAM BARS

120g (4¼oz) dark chocolate (made with
70–100% cacao)
120g (4¼oz) desiccated coconut
3 tbsp cold extra virgin coconut oil
1 tbsp honey (or agave syrup)
pinch of ground vanilla, or seeds of half
a vanilla pod

Makes 8 pieces 4 x 4 x 3cm (1½ x 1½ x 1¼in)

You will need a rectangular glass dish, 4 x 12cm (1½ x 5in), lined with baking
parchment. Make sure the edges of the paper hang over the sides.

Break the chocolate into pieces and put it in a bowl. Heat a saucepan of water over
a gentle heat and set the bowl over the water, making sure the water doesn't touch
the chocolate. Stir the chocolate occasionally, until melted.

While the chocolate is melting, whizz the coconut, coconut oil, honey and vanilla
in a blender. Transfer to a bowl, then work the mixture with your hands, until you
have a more sticky texture. You could add a little more coconut oil if necessary.

Using your hands, press the coconut mixture into the lined dish, so you have a
flat layer of coconut mixture.

Carefully pour the melted chocolate over the coconut, and leave to cool in the fridge
for at least 2 hours. After 1 hour, lightly score the chocolate with the tip of a sharp
knife – this will make it easier to cut into precise pieces once cooled.

When cool and firm, remove the coconut chocolate from the dish by inserting
a knife around the edges and lifting the baking parchment. Cut into bars or break
into large pieces. *Enjoy!*

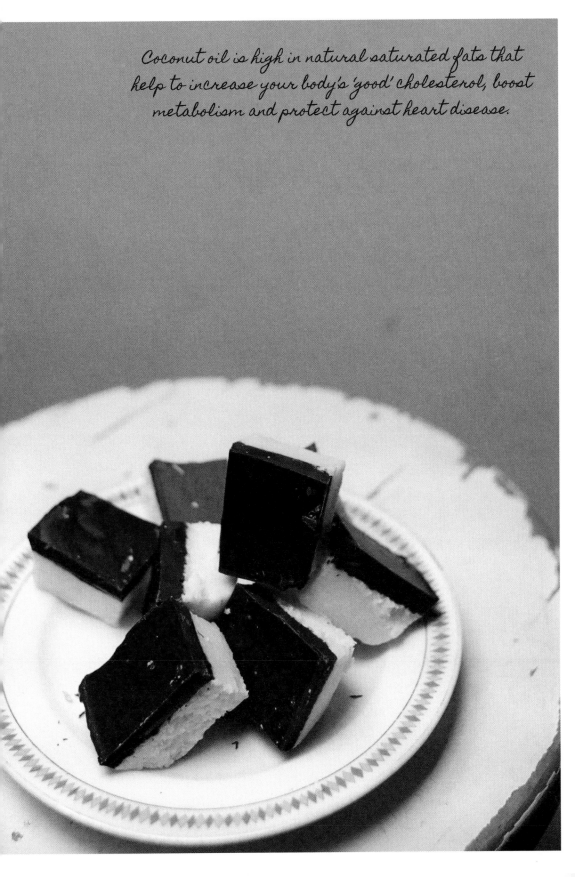

Coconut oil is high in natural saturated fats that help to increase your body's 'good' cholesterol, boost metabolism and protect against heart disease.

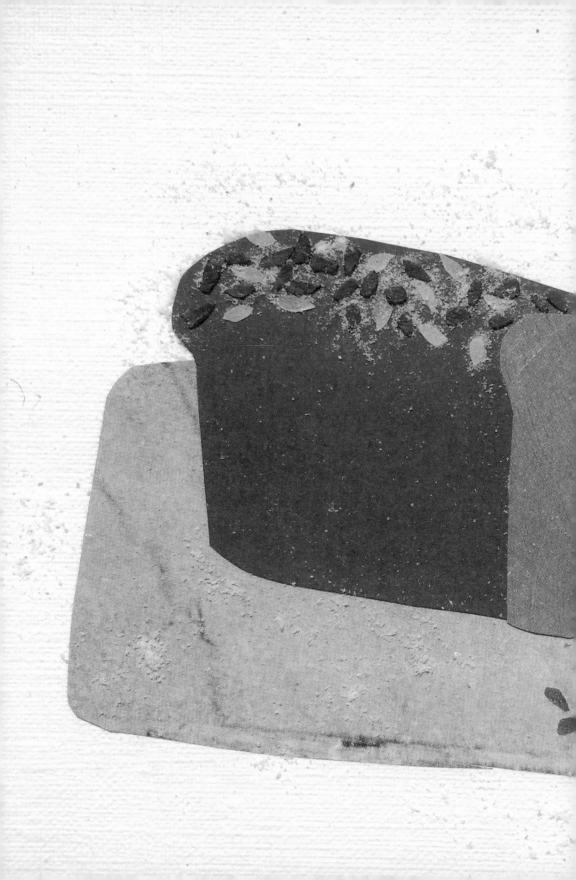

BREAD

Baking and experimenting with new ingredients
doesn't just give you a pleasant eating experience;
it also gives you new ideas and the inspiration
to use different types of grain in your kitchen.

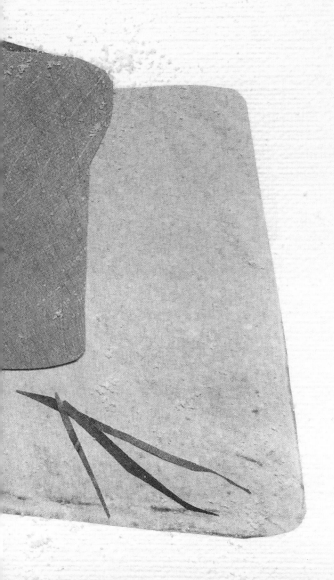

WHAT IS GLUTEN?

Gluten is the protein found in wheat flours (durum, emmer, spelt, farina, kamut, rye, barley and so on). It acts like a glue, helping bread and cakes to maintain their shape and structure. The same properties interfere with the breakdown and absorption of nutrients, including the nutrients from other foods in the same meal.

WHAT'S UP WITH GLUTEN FREE?

Through my work, as well as from my own experience, I have noticed that gluten intolerance is very common, and can cause fatigue, muscle weakness and digestive problems. Working as a nutritional therapist to improve the health of my clients in different ways, I found that, every time, they would feel better when they excluded gluten from their diet. There are many studies on this subject, and I have read and followed professionals in this area – such as Dr Mark Hyman, Dr Mercola, Tom O'Bryan – and they all talk about the same thing.

I want this book to be accessible to everyone, so I decided to include only gluten-free recipes (some of the recipes contain oats, which you could easily substitute if you are intolerant to them).

Important to add is that modern wheat is very different from ancient wheat. The proportion of gluten to protein has increased enormously as a result of hybridization. Additionally, until the nineteenth century, wheat was usually mixed with other grains, beans and nuts; it's only during the last two hundred years that the pure wheat flour has been milled into refined white flour.

THINK POSITIVE, ALWAYS!

Whatever you believe or decide, remember that there are so many foods in the world – and many natural gluten-free foods – that you might not have discovered yet. I am not against – nor religious about – any diet; I believe that everyone is different and needs to discover their own way of eating and enjoying food. Some people can handle gluten better than others.

The following are naturally gluten free: quinoa, amaranth, rice, buckwheat, millet, teff, maize, lentils, beans, chickpeas. Below is some useful information about the origins and the health properties of some of these ingredients.

Amaranth
• Originating in the Americas, this was a staple food of the Aztecs, Incas and Mayans.
• High in minerals like potassium, iron, phosphorus, calcium, magnesium and manganese, as well as proteins and fibres.

- Known to help prevent health conditions such as diabetes and heart disease, support good stomach health and lower hypertension.

Buckwheat
- Related to sorrel, knotweed and rhubarb, buckwheat was first cultivated in Southeast Asia and then spread to the Middle East and Europe.
- A naturally gluten-free grain with high levels of B vitamins, vitamin E, chromium, copper, magnesium, iron, zinc, flavonoids and fibres.
- Very gentle on the stomach, which helps the bowels. High in antioxidants, with anti-inflammatory properties.

Lentils
- Grown throughout the world, primarily coming from Canada, India, Turkey and Australia.
- A good source of essential amino acids, and especially vitamins and minerals like vitamin B_1 and folate, copper and magnesium.
- Supports brain function and maintains enzyme production which is essential for energy. Promotes healing.

Millet
- Widely grown around the world, this small-seeded grass is very popular in Asia and Africa and has its origin in tropical western Africa.
- Contains a good amount of magnesium, iron, potassium and B vitamins.
- Easy to digest, and good for metabolism and heart health.

Quinoa
- The quinoa plant grows in the highland plains of the Andes, but can also be found in Europe.
- High in protein, with all the essential amino acids that the human body needs. Also a good source of B vitamins, vitamin E, and also essential minerals like folate, iron, copper, calcium, potassium and magnesium.
- Good for intestine and gut health and balancing cholesterol levels. Its powerful antioxidants protect from harmful free radicals, infections and ageing. A great source of vegetable protein that strengthens muscles and provides long-lasting energy.

Rice
- Native to Asia and certain parts of Africa. Now cultivated all around the world.
- Rich in all B vitamins and magnesium.
- Rice is gentle on the stomach, anti-inflammatory and calming. Supports metabolism and promotes healthy hair and skin.

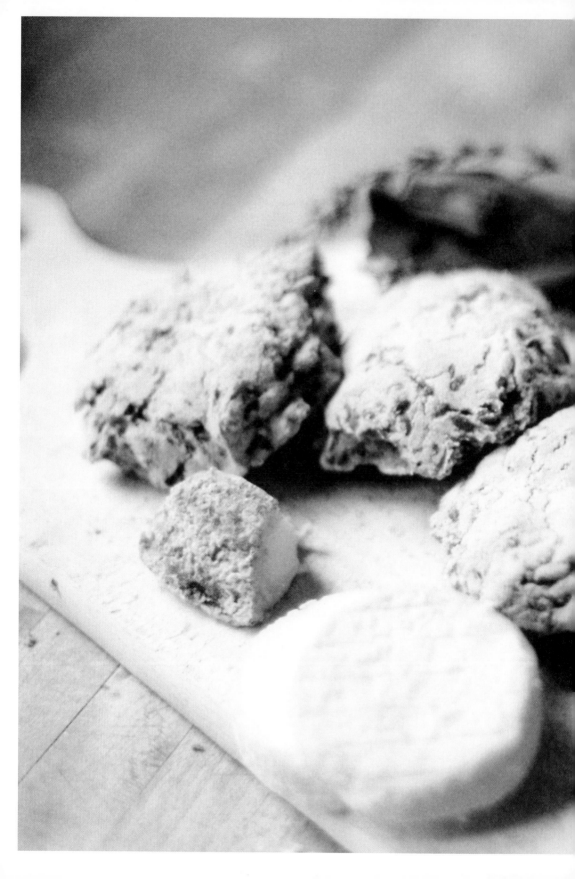

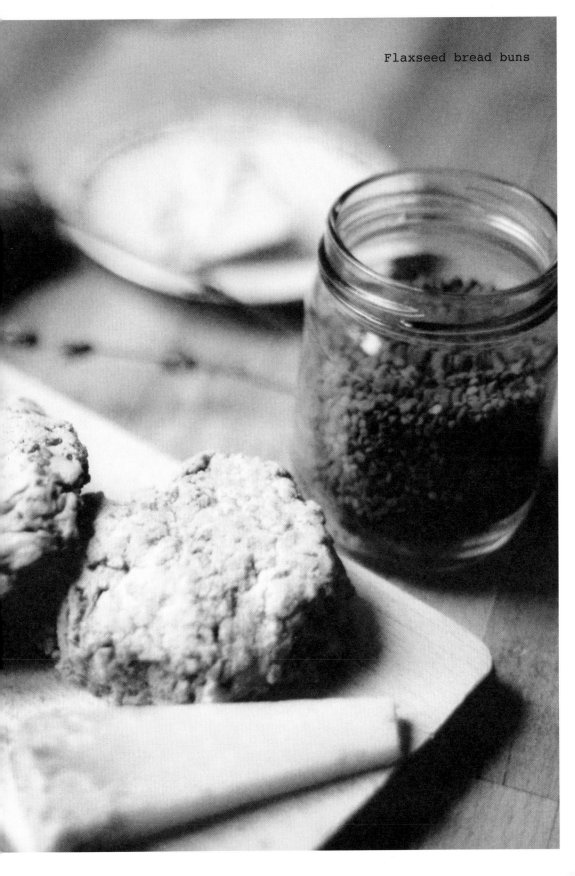

FLAXSEED BREAD BUNS

70g (2¼oz) flaxseeds
200ml (7floz) water
120g (4¼oz) buckwheat flour, plus 50g (1¾oz)
for kneading
200g (7oz) rice flour
2 tsp baking powder
1 tsp salt
1 tsp extra virgin coconut oil
200ml (7floz) water
1 tsp ground cinnamon

Makes 6 buns

Soak the flaxseeds in the water for 2 hours.

Preheat the oven to 185°C/365°F/Gas 5 and grease a baking sheet.

Add the dry ingredients to the soaked flaxseed mixture, then pour in the coconut oil (if it's solid, warm it up in the oven for a few seconds to melt it) and 100ml (3½fl oz) of the water. Mix everything together, then add the remaining water. The dough should be very sticky. It should also be brown-grey in colour, as buckwheat is naturally grey – this is normal.

Weigh out the 50g (1¾oz) buckwheat flour for kneading, then coat your hands in some of the flour and knead the dough. Divide the dough into 6 buns. Each one should weigh about 130–140g (around 4¾oz).

Place the buns on the baking sheet and bake in the middle of the oven for 20–30 minutes.

MULTIGRAIN BREAD

150g (5oz) almonds
100g (3½oz) sesame seeds
100g (3½oz) flaxseeds
100g (3½oz) sunflower seeds
150g (5oz) pumpkin seeds
2 tbsp extra virgin olive oil
1 tsp ground ginger
1 tsp ground cinnamon
pinch of salt
5 eggs, beaten

Makes 1 loaf

Preheat the oven to 160°C/320°F/Gas 3. Grease a 450g (1lb) loaf tin with coconut oil or line with baking parchment, leaving the edges hanging over the sides of the tin.

In a KitchenAid or blender, whizz the almonds until you have a fine flour. Add the other seeds and mix to combine. Pour in the oil, then stir in the spices and salt.

Add the beaten eggs to the mixture, combine well, then pour into the loaf tin.

Bake in the middle of the oven for 1 hour 15 minutes, then leave to cool in the tin before serving.

If you wish, you could add some poppy seeds before transferring the mixture to the loaf tin.

Naturally gluten-free bread that is high in protein and fibre. I assure you this will fill a hungry belly!

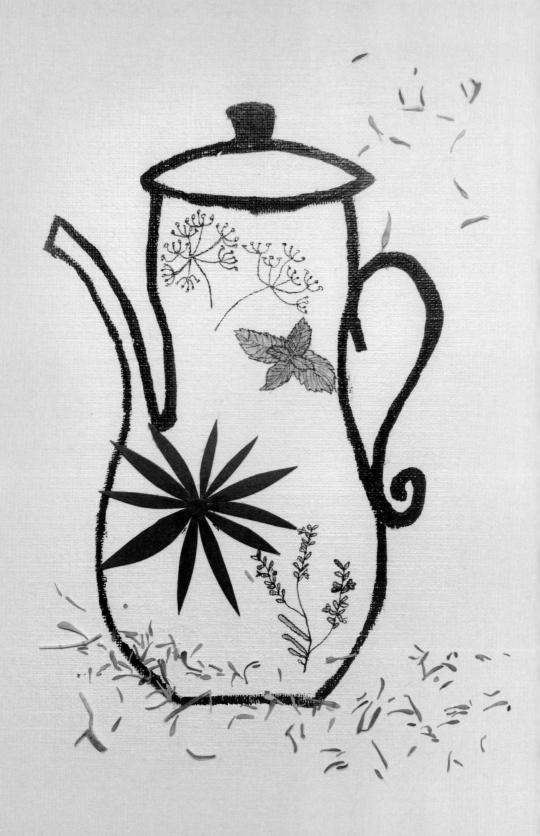

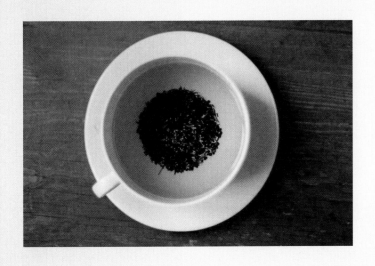

HERBAL TEAS
& HOT DRINKS

My sense of intuition and sensitivity for body and soul is strong, and this is something I make use of in the kitchen and as a nutritional therapist. And the power of herbal remedies – here, in the form of teas – should never be underestimated!

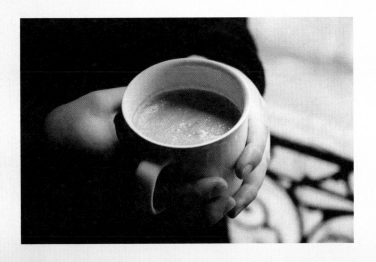

The oldest and most commonly applied medicinal practice in the world today is the use of herbal remedies. I have tremendous respect for the power of plants. The parts usually used for medicinal purposes are the seeds, berries, roots, leaves, bark or flowers. Today, you can find capsules, tinctures or even use the dried plant for infusions.

I strongly believe that if we could go back to a more natural approach to medicine the world would be better off. In this day and age, the use of chemical drugs is surprisingly high and I am sceptical as to whether it makes people feel much better. Chemical drugs usually treat acute symptoms, but don't address the root of the problem. I long for a world in which we respect the power of nature and, with the help of our intuition, practise care towards it.

It's important to identify what is good for each individual: every*thing* is not good for every*one*. No matter what the scientific benefits of any given plant may be, we are all different and need to be regarded as unique.

Having studied the many different herbs, my diploma in phytotherapy helped me use those herbs in practice. Here, I share some of my favourite plants; they are easy to find and are commonly used for their health benefits. And you may well be surprised to find that you already have some of these plants in your home …

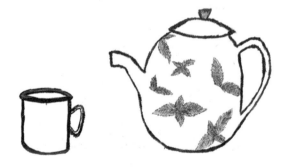

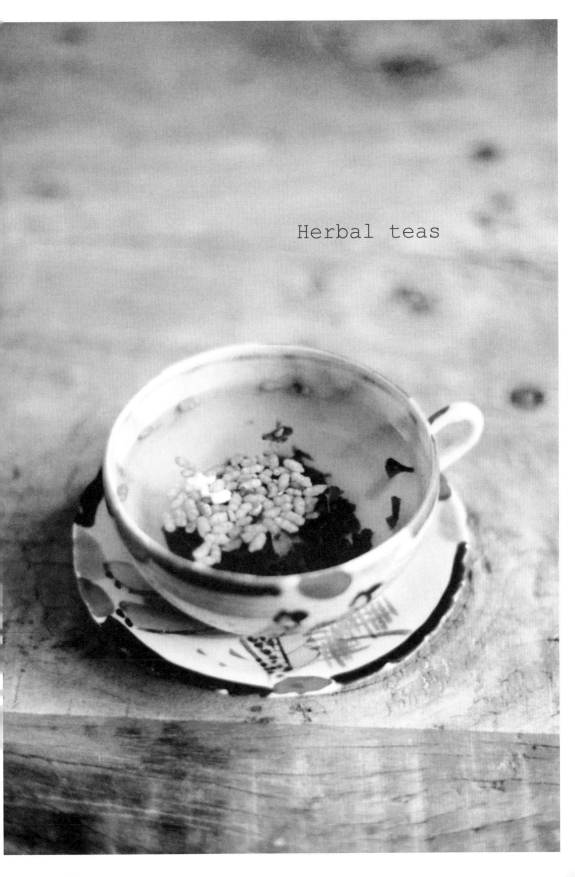

Herbal teas

MAKING YOUR HERBAL INFUSION

- Choose your dried herbs or plants.
- Boil 1 litre (around 2 pints) of water in a kettle or on the stove.
- When it reaches a rolling boil, pour the water into your teapot.
- Take your herbs (see beneficial properties and doses listed below) and place them in the water, then let it stand for 10 minutes. This usually produces a good, strong infusion. If you leave it for longer, you will get a stronger tea, but if you prefer it weaker, infuse for a shorter time.
- Strain the infusion through a strainer into a mug, or filter it into a flask and keep it to drink during the day.

Cardamom

This spice contains many essential oils and has antiseptic, digestive and diuretic health benefits. Can boost metabolism and aid circulation.
Dosage: 10 green cardamom pods

Chamomile

Known for its calming and cramp-relieving properties. Can help with stomach ache, menstrual cramps and sleeping problems. Also good for digestion.
Dosage: 4—8g

Dandelion

A diuretic herb that can support the liver and the kidneys. It has a bitter taste and helps the digestion.
Dosage: 4—8g

Fennel seeds

Great as a digestive aid and to relieve cramps, gas and bloating. Promotes oral hygiene and can alleviate bad breath.
Dosage: 1 tbsp

Ginger

Fabulous for circulation, digestion and to increase libido. A strong antioxidant that can boost the immune system.
Dosage: about 8g fresh ginger, peeled and chopped

Milk thistle

A powerful plant, commonly used to protect the liver. It is a strong antioxidant that aids the detoxification of the liver.
Dosage: 4g

Pau d'arco — my favourite

A bark from the huge trees of the Amazon rainforest and other tropical parts of Latin America. It has long been used in herbal medicine all over the world. Pau d'arco contains flavonoids and is an astringent. It has antibacterial, antiviral and antifungal properties and supports the lymphatic system – and is therefore very effective when used as part of a detox. It cleans the blood, strengthens the immune system and promotes good digestion. Used traditionally for gastrointestinal problems, candida and yeast infections, constipation and allergies, among other complaints.
Dosage: 1½ tbsp

Peppermint

Aids digestion and can relieve stomach pain; peppermint is a cooling herb that can help reduce stress and boost energy levels. The aroma of peppermint has been shown to enhance memory and increase alertness.
Dosage: 4g

Rosemary

Boosts circulation and aids the memory. Rosemary can relieve headaches and migraine, aid digestion and fight muscle inflammation.
Dosage: 4g

Thyme

Contains essential oils like thymol, which has been scientifically found to be antifungal and antiseptic. Has one of the highest antioxidant levels among herbs. Good for coughs, sore throat and inflammation. Can also relieve bronchial cramps.
Dosage: 4g

Valerian

A popular alternative remedy for sleeping problems. Also known to ease tension and anxiety, and can calm an upset stomach, headache and other stress-related issues.
Note: Valerian can interact with some medications, so always speak to your doctor to see if valerian is right for you.
Dosage: 1–4g

This information is general and the dosages given are suggestions only. Always speak to your doctor or nutritional therapist before using any of these remedies.

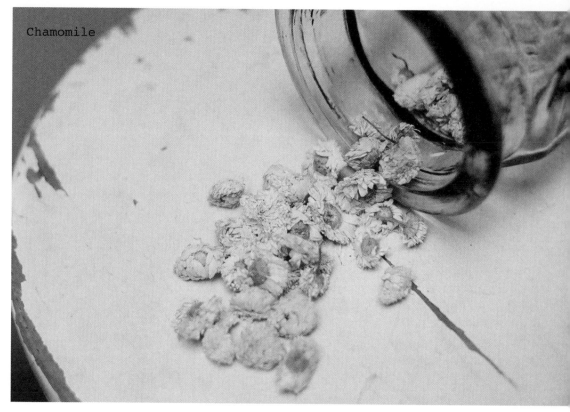

Chamomile

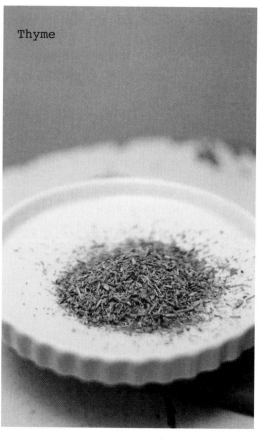

Thyme

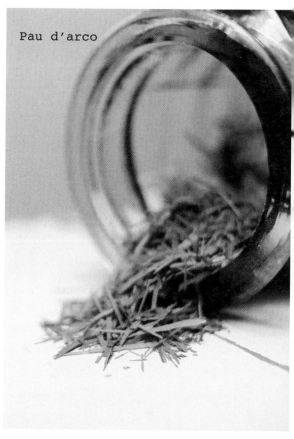

Pau d'arco

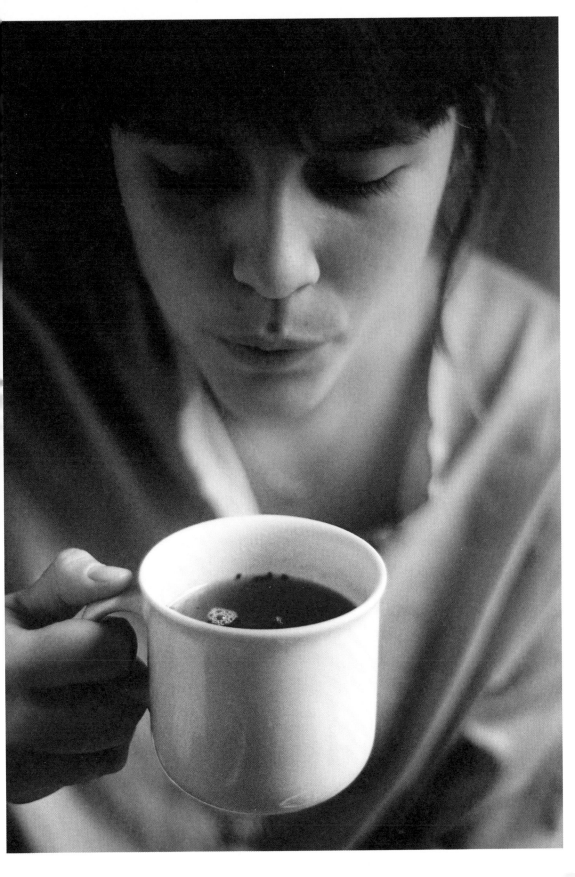

CALMING CHAI

1 vanilla pod
4 green cardamom pods
1 cinnamon stick
3 cloves
1cm (⅓in) piece fresh root ginger, thinly sliced
600ml (1 pint) filtered water
small handful of chamomile flowers
100ml (3½floz) almond milk (you can make your
own — see page 25 — or buy unsweetened)
2 tbsp honey (optional)

Makes about 700ml (24fl oz)

Split the vanilla pod in two and scrape out the seeds. You can use both parts in the infusion, depending on how strong you want the vanilla flavour to be.

Set a saucepan over a medium heat, add the cardamom pods and gently cook for a few minutes to enhance the flavours.

Add the vanilla seeds and pod (if using), cinnamon stick, cloves and ginger, and pour over the water. Bring to the boil, then reduce the heat to low and infuse for 10 minutes. Add the chamomile flowers and infuse for another 5 minutes.

Pour the infusion through a tea strainer to remove the spices (if you wish), then pour back into the pan.

Add the almond milk and heat through. Serve with some honey, or just as it is.

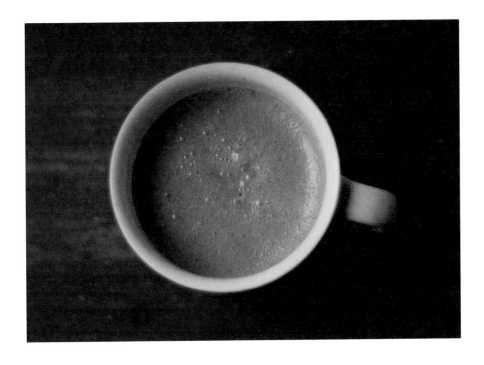

MY HOMEMADE HOT CHOCOLATE

50ml (2floz) water
200ml (7floz) coconut milk
4 small pieces of 100% organic chocolate
1 tsp maca powder
pinch of ground vanilla
1 tsp organic honey (or agave syrup)

Makes 1 big cup of hot chocolate

Heat the water until it's almost boiling, then add the coconut milk, chocolate, maca and vanilla. Reduce the heat to low, and stir until the chocolate is melted.

Serve in a cup with some honey.

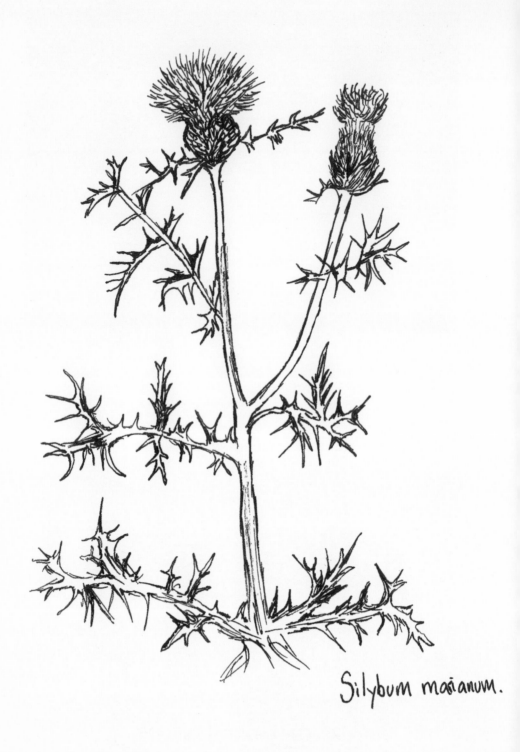

Silybum marianum.

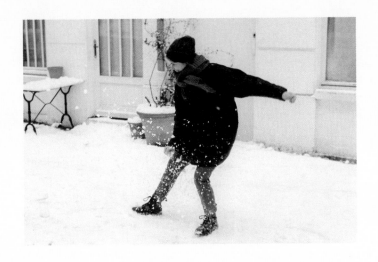

BODY & SOUL DETOX

By detox, I mean 'clean up'. Everything needs to
be cleaned once in a while, even the environment
inside the human body. I want to share with
you my knowledge and experience – along with
some simple tools – of keeping your inner and
outer body clean. And remember: feeding your
mind and your spirit, and enjoying life, is just
as important as feeding your body.

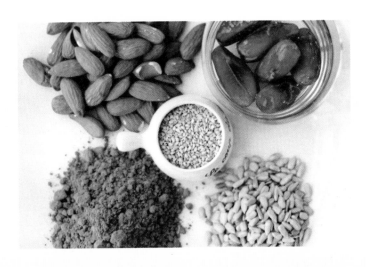

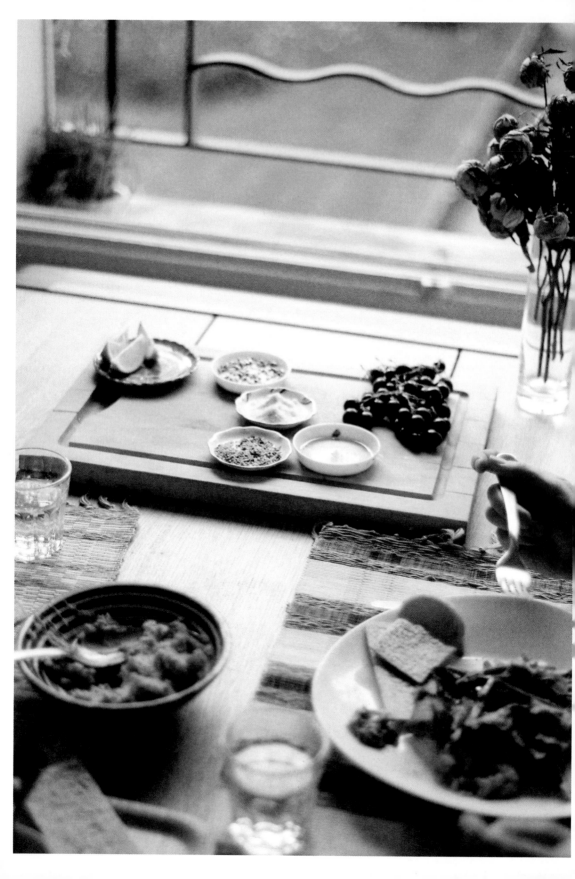

CONSCIOUS EATING

Meals on the run, TV dinners, eating while working – sadly, these are all too common in our lives today. We rarely have time to relax before, during or after a meal.

We forget that, when eating, we are supporting our bodies with nutrition and energy, and digestion is a big part of that, because it is through this process that we are able to absorb necessary vitamins, minerals and trace elements. If we rush through eating our lunch, there is no chance for proper digestion to take place, as the process doesn't work efficiently under stress.

The parasympathetic nervous system takes care of (among other things) the digestion, while the sympathetic nervous system is associated with stress; both systems work together and are two main parts of the autonomic nervous system. Because these two integral systems are so connected, for optimal digestion we need to eliminate stress and other distractions at mealtimes.

Advice for conscious eating:
- Clear your eating space – remove any distractions.
- Enjoy your food – be aware of the taste, texture, temperature and smell.
- Skipping meals, eating a low-calorie diet or having imbalanced meals all lead to nutrient deficiencies that can give rise to compulsive or binge eating.
- Mindfulness and routine: when you're mindful of your meal, you enjoy it more, and when you have a routine and don't snack all the time, your meal will feel more precious and important. Constant light snacking disturbs the digestion, and can easily lead to mood swings, gassiness and bad eating habits.

Advice for optimal digestion:
- Soaking grains, seeds and nuts activates the enzymes in the food, making digestion easier.
- Chew your food sufficiently!
- Remove stresses from your environment.
- Stick to a routine.
- Eat dinner at least 2 hours before going to bed.
- Drink herbal teas such as dandelion, fennel, licorice, green tea, ginger, chamomile, lapacho …

SENSIBLE DETOXING

We live in a hectic environment, full of pollution from traffic and other sources, and we are constantly exposed to toxins and chemicals, parasites and bacteria, that our bodies absorb and have to deal with. On top of that, research has shown that our water contains potentially harmful toxins such as arsenic, fluoride and chlorine, among others.

The particles from these toxins can become lodged in our bodies, which is detrimental to our inner well-being, both physically and mentally.

If you feel tired, have irritated skin or feel bloated after meals, a 5-day cleanse could make you feel revitalized and full of energy.

Given how hard our body works for us every single minute of every day, I think it deserves a rest and some tender loving care a couple of times a year!

So, what does a clean diet mean?
- Avoid refined flour, sugar and processed foods.
- Cut out caffeine.
- Avoid alcohol.
- Balance your blood sugar by eating protein such as protein shakes, eggs and nut butters for breakfast.
- Eat regularly throughout the day and don't skip meals.
- Don't eat within 3 hours of bedtime.
- Cut out dairy products and consider eliminating other common allergens such as gluten.
- Increase the fibre in your diet, from vegetables, fruit, nuts, seeds, beans and whole grains.
- Increase your levels of omega-3 fats by eating more oily fish such as sardines, herring and wild salmon, as well as omega-3 eggs and walnuts.
- Eat organic food, especially when it comes animal products, to avoid environmental oestrogens from pesticides.

How to approach a detox
There are different types of detox. You can go for a daily detox routine, which is simple, cheap and not too intense, but very important in the long term. Or, you can go for a more intense approach, with stricter conditions. The most common time frame for a detox programme seems to be 5 to 10 days.

The best time of year to do an intense cleanse is spring or autumn, as the temperature is more mellow – neither very hot nor very cold – and it prepares us for the next season.

A detox always needs to be undertaken carefully, seriously and safely. We can't know all the toxins and bacteria lurking deep in our bodies, and, when they are released, we need to be sure that they are flushed out without causing us harm. People often start too hard; herbs are powerful, so it's important to be sensible (bear in mind that headaches and tiredness are common in the first few days).

It is important to get the process right, to eliminate unwanted bacteria and support the liver, which needs to work to take care of everything else. I would say there are three steps to follow in your routine:

Cleaning
- First of all, take a look at your diet. Add lots of natural, nutrition-rich and colourful foods and cut out the less healthy ones (see opposite).
- Choose a cleansing herb to take throughout your detox – for example pau d'arco, chlorella or artemesia annu.

Diuretics
- Add a diuretic herb – for example, dandelion, flaxseed or celery – to support the elimination of the bacteria from your body. Don't forget to drink lots of filtered water.
- Add going for a sauna to your detox programme, as sweating is another great way to flush out those toxins (see below).

Antioxidants and liver support
- Supporting your body is a very important part of this process. Choose good, healthy foods and supplement them with spices like cayenne pepper, turmeric, ginger and black pepper.
- Milk thistle, artichoke and dandelion are good herbs to include.

It is important that you read any instructions carefully. Always consult your doctor or nutritional therapist if you have any concerns.

Skin
The skin is made up of nerves, glands and cell layers that, when healthy, protect the body from extreme temperatures and chemicals. It's the body's largest organ and plays a crucial role in supporting optimal detoxification.

Sauna
Many gyms have saunas and, as well as giving you a very nice warm feeling, these help you to eliminate toxins. If you exercise before having a sauna, gently dry brushing your body (see below) will help further elimination.

Dry brushing
Dry brushing is my personal favourite. It stimulates the lymphatic system, removes dead dry skin, clears clogged pores and increases the circulation. You will need a high-quality brush, made with natural materials. Brush daily for best results – try to incorporate it into your daily routine. Before your morning shower is a good time (avoid brushing just before bed, as it may leave you feeling energized, and not ready for sleep!).

Always brush towards your heart, as this is best for circulation and the lymphatic system. The entire body can be brushed, with the exception of the face (unless you have a special brush designed for delicate skin), genitals and any areas with irritations or abrasions. The pressure should be firm, but not painful – don't scrub.

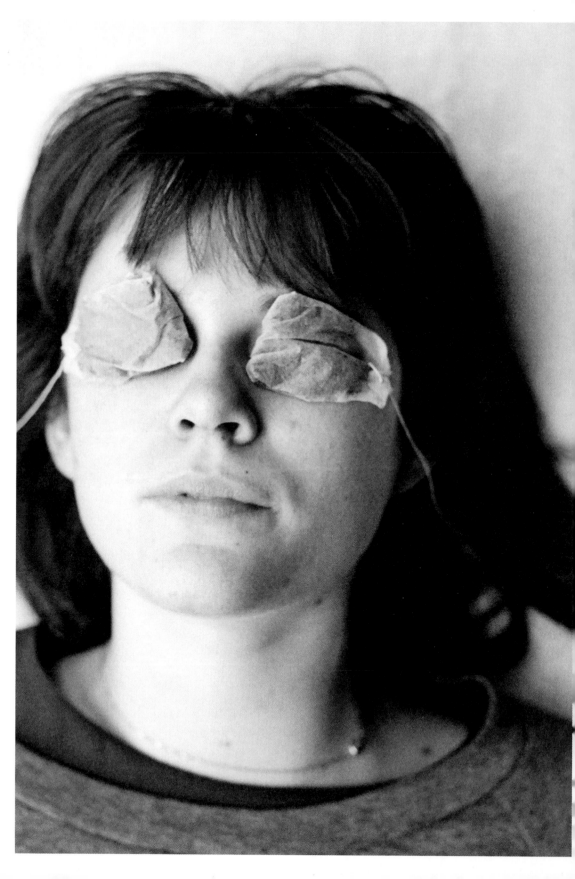

Herbs for daily or intensive detox

Pau d'arco
A bark that is drunk as a tea or taken as a herbal tincture or powder. Very effective against viruses, bacteria and parasites. Also cleans the lymphatic system and the blood.

Dandelion
Dandelion is great taken in the morning with freshly squeezed lemon juice, to boost liver and kidney function. It is also a diuretic and is very beneficial for the digestion. Good combined with a cleansing herb.

Protease enzymes
These enzymes break down the protein in your food; this occurs naturally, and there are also supplements available which can be taken between meals to help the body break down old proteins that can cause inflammation. They also eliminate bacteria and parasites.

Cascara
A laxative herb that supports the thyroid function. Should not be used for prolonged periods, and take great care not to take too much.

Oregano
Used as a natural antibiotic, as it is antibacterial and kills viruses.

Artemisia annua
Also known as sweet wormwood, this herb has been used in Chinese medicine and also in other parts of Asia for many thousands of years, to target parasites. Can be useful when cleansing the system, and especially for those travelling to foreign regions that their body (and, therefore, their bacteria) may not be used to.

Ginger
Not only is ginger good for circulation and inflammation, it is also a strong antioxidant and gives you energy and strength.

For further information and recommendations, please see your nutritional therapist.

NATURAL RADIANTS

Facial wash

Natural oils are fantastic for use as a facial wash, removing make-up and leaving the skin smooth, clean and moisturized without any additives or other perfumes or chemicals. Make sure you get an organic quality oil. Choose one that suits you best (see below), and get started!

Instructions

Place an almond-sized drop of oil in your hands and apply to your face and neck, then gently pat the skin with a cotton pad to wipe away any excess oil. Alternatively, pour the oil directly onto the cotton pad and use it to remove any dirt and make-up.

You can even use the oil to remove mascara; just be careful not to get it in your eyes, or it could sting.

Suitable oils

Almond A classic 'beauty' oil that is very gentle and suits many people, with a natural smell and smooth feeling.
Coconut Antibacterial and can be used on more problematic skin.
Olive A bit thicker in consistency; beneficial for dry skin. Very readily available.
Apricot Good for ageing and sensitive skin.
Avocado Beneficial for sensitive, 'tired' and dry skin.
Sesame Good for dry skin; can be mixed with almond or other oil – the fragrance of sesame oil is pretty strong!

Honey mask

Honey is calming, nourishing and moisturizing for your skin. Always use a raw, organic honey – preferably a locally sourced one.

Instructions

Take 1–2 teaspoons of honey in your fingers and gently massage it over your face and neck, avoiding the area around your eyes. Leave the honey on your skin for 15–20 minutes, then wash your face with warm water to rinse it all off (you can finish off with a cotton pad to make sure it's all removed). If you like, apply some natural oil afterwards. Now you're ready for a good night's sleep!

Facial scrub

Coconut oil and brown sugar make a nice and easy homemade facial scrub, to remove dead skin cells and blackheads.

Instructions

Simply mix equal parts of the oil and sugar – you can make a big batch and store it in a glass jar in your bathroom. Gently massage the mixture into your face, using a small circular motion with your fingers, then wash it off with warm water. As with the honey mask, you can follow the scrub with your choice of natural oil, to moisturize your face.

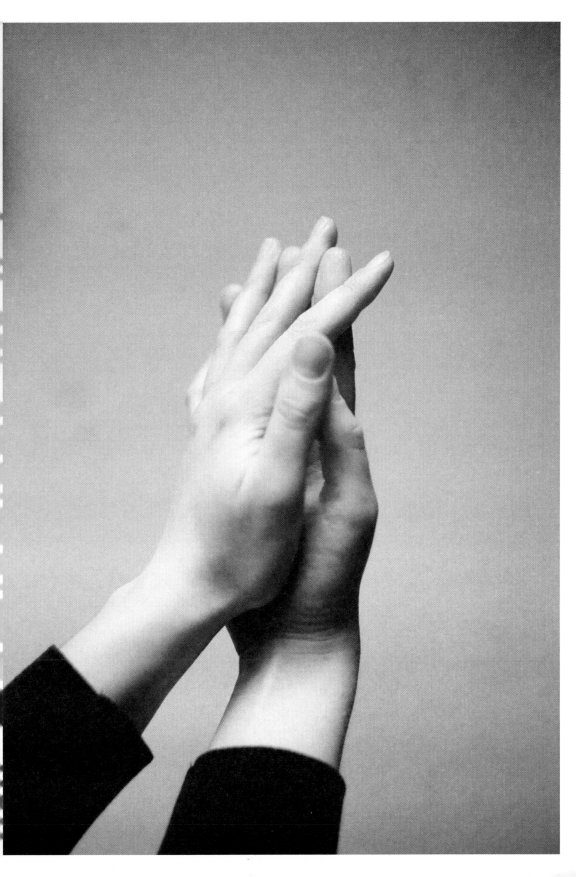

Shaving — unisex

Oils are great for getting a smooth shave, and can be used as an alternative to shaving creams. Shea butter makes a great aftershave lotion, and coconut oil can be used to discourage breakouts caused by shaving. Both can be applied after shaving.

Instructions

To make your own shaving cream, mix 1.5 tablespoons coconut oil, 2 tablespoons shea butter and 1 tablespoon olive oil. Whisk for a few minutes until the mixture takes on a more fluffy consistency. Then it's ready to use!

Sleep

To relax and reset we need to sleep, preferably for 7 to 9 hours every night. The body produces the highest quantity of growth hormone during the deepest stages of sleep. This aids cell and tissue repair. Collagen, a protein that keeps skin strong and elastic, is also produced while we sleep.

During the night is also the time for the liver to detoxify. A lack of sleep will not only affect liver detoxification; as many studies show, it also has a considerable impact on the immune system, mental health and hormonal balance.

So, sleep is a vital natural radiant, and is as important as eating well and exercise.

FOODS

Nuts

The antioxidants found in nuts – especially almonds – are very beneficial for the skin. Vitamin E fights free radicals and also helps the skin retain moisture.

Red & green vegetables

Orange and red vegetables are full of beta-carotene. The body converts beta-carotene into vitamin A, which prevents cell damage and premature ageing. Spinach, rocket and other green leafy vegetables provide lots of vitamin A, too.

Vitamin C (citrus fruits)

Vitamin C is necessary for the production of collagen, the protein that forms the basic structure of your skin.

Probiotics

Probiotics are widely known for their beneficial role in the health of the gut, but their benefits are not only limited to the digestive tract. Research has shown how probiotics can help with skin conditions like dryness, improve collagen and stabilize the microflora in your skin, helping with irritation. For example, eczema is more than just a skin problem; it signals problems with the immune system and, in fact, is said to be one of the first signs of allergy when found in newborns.

'There are about 100 trillion microorganisms – bacteria, fungi and more – living on and in your body. The bacterial cells also outnumber human cells by 10 to 1. Even after you wash, there are still 1 million bacteria living on every square centimeter of your skin.

In other words, the bacteria living on your skin are involved in a symbiotic relationship with you. The bacteria on your inner elbow, for instance, process the raw fats it produces and in turn moisturize your skin.' DR MERCOLA

So, having balanced, good gut flora will give you healthy skin.

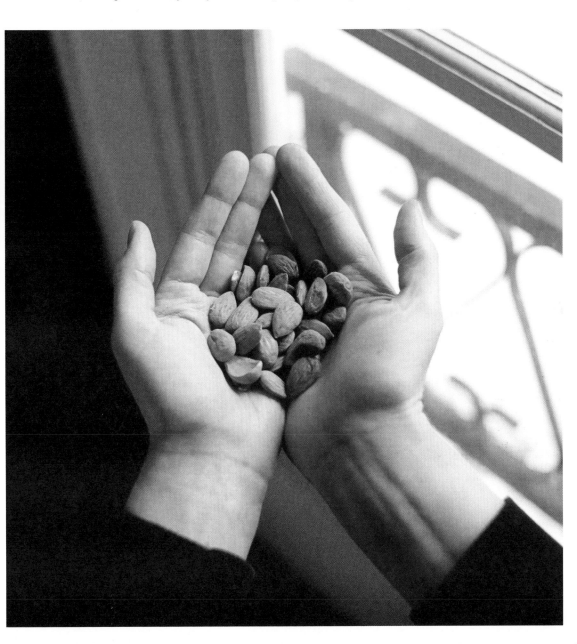

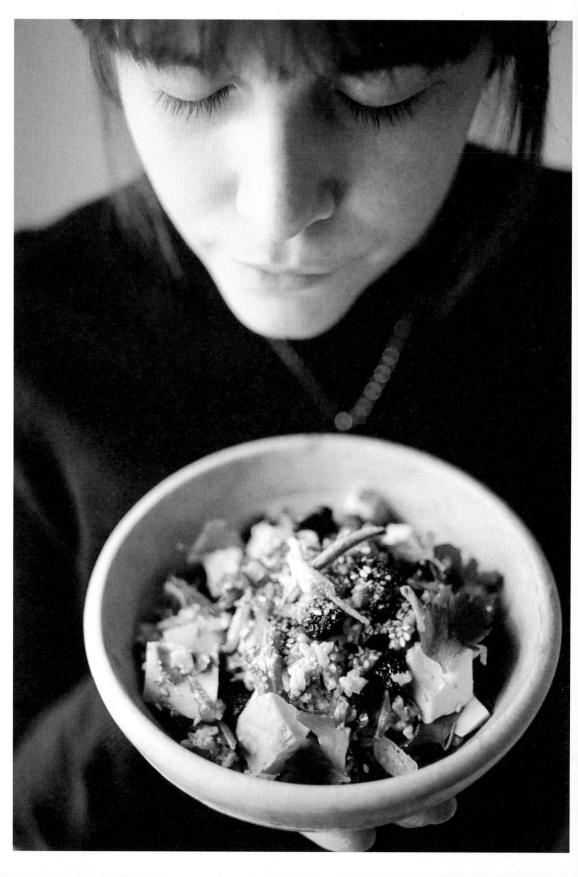

HEALTHY MIND, HEALTHY GUT

I wanted to include this section because 'being healthy', today, is often just about eating right, but not much about enjoying the simple, beautiful life itself. I see how this approach causes a lot of unnecessary and unhealthy stress for many people – and it's time to address this imbalance. I am not promoting a certain religion or diet; I simply believe in the power of the individual, and in the positive and honest mind.

For example, the word 'diet' is a strong word. If you ask me what diet I have, I would say I eat what I like, want and feel like eating in the moment. If I were to use one word, maybe something like 'qualitarian' would describe it quite well – fresh, organic, seasonal, colourful, quality food, made with care. I love trying new dishes, having home-cooked dinners made by a loved one. I enjoy eating fish when I am at the coast in Barcelona with my Spanish family, as well as eating my mum's lentil stew on a cold day in Sweden.

If I eat too much bread I feel that I lose my energy, and if I don't get my veggies I feel tired. I know my body, and I know that if I eat what's good for me, my gut and my mind are happy.

THE SECOND BRAIN

The stomach, technically known as the enteric nervous system, is our second brain. There are sheaths of neurons embedded in the walls of the long tube of the alimentary canal, which measures about 9m (30ft) from the oesophagus to the anus. The second brain contains some 100 million neurons, which is more than in the spinal cord or the peripheral nervous system.

One of the neurons present in the gut produces neurotransmitters like serotonin, also found in the brain. Serotonin is involved in mood control, depression and aggression and, in fact, the greatest concentration of serotonin is found in the intestines, not the brain.

We all know the feeling of butterflies in the stomach; it signals a part of our physiological stress response. It's likely that the nerves in the gut have a big influence on our emotions.

The reason why stress and other emotions can contribute to gastrointestinal symptoms is because the brain sends signals to your gut. And, according to a study published in the journal *Gastroenterology*, these signals also travel the opposite way, from gut to brain.

Gut bacteria are vulnerable to our diet and lifestyle; about 80 per cent of the immune system is located here. Nurturing and supporting the gut with healthy bacteria such as the probiotics found in yogurt and fermented food is important for optimal health.

What you eat will affect your mood, and how you feel will affect your appetite; it all works together. It's common knowledge, for example, that many additives, preservatives and food colourants can cause behavioural changes, as does sugar. Numerous studies have explored the links between high-sugar diets and mental health conditions such as depression and schizophrenia. Having a high-sugar diet doesn't only cause mood changes, but also poor nutrition.

There is no doubt that the mind and the gut have a big impact on one another.

MEDITATION & MINDFULNESS

When it comes to a healthy mind, being able to feel, and be aware of, what your body needs takes some practice, but it doesn't require much if you consider what it will give you in return.

To be aware of the present moment is mindfulness

The practice of meditation is associated with a sense of peacefulness and physical relaxation, but studies also show that it provides cognitive and psychological benefits, and that meditation literally alters your brain. People who practise meditation, yoga or mindfulness live a happier, less stressful life.

When you disconnect, and listen to your breathing, something very profound is happening. Breathing is life energy, and when you focus just on the sound and flow of breathing and let everything else go, you not only relax and become calm but you also let your life energy flow and your spiritual mind grow.

My experience, and how I got hooked on yoga and meditation

I have always loved exercising in a variety of forms – dancing, boxing, running, to name but a few. In 2009, after coming home from an extended trip to Australia and New Zealand, where I bumped into a number of people who practised yoga, I decided to give it a try.

I remember the first class so well. I was feeling restless, stiff (even though I was already quite flexible, thanks to the dancing), and I was almost getting irritated by the 'zen' ambience of the teacher. After 90 minutes of vinyasa practice, it was time for shavasana – the meditation. The teacher guided us, and I remember coming into a very deep, relaxing state that I had never really experienced before. Everything was quiet, calm and beautiful, and I didn't feel restless any more.